I0480327

MEDICAL INDUSTRIAL COMPLEX

The $ickness Industry, Big Pharma and Suppressed Cures

THE UNDERGROUND KNOWLEDGE SERIES

James&Lance
MORCAN

MEDICAL INDUSTRIAL COMPLEX: THE $ICKNESS INDUSTRY, BIG PHARMA AND SUPPRESSED
CURES

Published by:

Sterling Gate Books
28 St. Heliers Place,
Papamoa 3118,
Bay of Plenty,
New Zealand

sterlinggatebooks@gmail.com

Special Note: This title is an extended version of Chapter 11 of *The Orphan Conspiracies: 29 Conspiracy Theories from The Orphan Trilogy* (Sterling Gate Books, 2014) by James Morcan & Lance Morcan. This title therefore contains a combination of new material as well as recycled material (in many cases verbatim excerpts) from *The Orphan Conspiracies*.

Publication data:

Morcan, James 1978-
Morcan, Lance 1948-
Title: Medical Industrial Complex: The $ickness Industry, Big Pharma and Suppressed Cures
Edition: First ed.
Format: Paperback
Publisher: Sterling Gate Books

TABLE OF CONTENTS

FOREWORD

This book is part of *The Underground Knowledge Series* by James & Lance Morcan. In it, they raise some very important questions concerning the state of modern medicine today and the major players in the highly profitable medical sector. Questions that certainly need to be brought out into the open and discussed with politicians and administrators who often hide behind closed doors.

While it would be nice to think none of the negative issues raised in this book are true, my suspicions are that, sadly, this is not the case.

In my own career as a pharmacist spanning 40 years, I have seen many examples of patients falling through the cracks in the health system as a direct result of health providers focusing on high patient turnover on a 'fee-for-service' basis with no guarantee of results.

On top of this, all too often health professionals have to work within systems created by politicians and administrators that allow for zero direct responsibility for patient outcomes. In fact, it is interesting to consider that, despite the millions of dollars invested in research, we have few medicines that actually *cure* patients in the real sense of the word.

Sadly, for many doctors, 'cure' means 'a quick fix,' often putting patients on a medicine for the rest of their lives with the possibility of adverse side effects, and no guarantee of a positive outcome. In light of this, there is no hiding the huge influence drug companies have on the practice of medicine which has stalled finding real cures.

The health system is more about the ambulance at the bottom of a cliff than a fence at the top. What we need, I believe, is a focus on real cures and prevention of disease with a strong focus on the body (healthy lifestyle), mind and spirit.

I am sure people want to take more responsibility for their health, but often do not know where to start. Equally, some health professionals do not take too kindly to patients who want to be involved in decisions about their treatment.

The Morcans highlight the tendency to label holistic as *quackery* – an ironic description when you consider holistic practitioners tend to focus on dealing with the causes of disease rather than just treating symptoms with medicines.

I am excited that more doctors today are practicing functional medicine, which has a lot in common with a holistic approach. Incidentally, I encourage people to spell holistic 'wholistic' to emphasise the whole (big) picture.

Serious questions need to be asked about a health 'system' in which politicians are often reluctant to invest money in long term, preventative measures. Measures that may take years to show a return on investment. Instead, they tend to focus on short term tangible things like spending more money to reduce waiting surgical waiting lists (to win votes) instead of dealing with the long term underlying causes, such as obesity, that are plaguing our world.

Regarding obesity, the public health message to reduce fat intake has actually led to many people getting their energy from high Glycaemic index carbohydrates. These often lead to insulin resistance, diabetes and, believe it or not, the production of fat in the body, giving rise to obesity, which is linked to many diseases including cancer.

Denis Toovey B. *App. Sc. (Pharmacy) and Post Grad. Dip. (Clinical Pharmacy)*
Retired Pharmacist and Author of *Better Health for You – An Insider's Big Picture Guide.*

INTRODUCTION

You don't need to be a genius to know that corruption is rife in the world's most lucrative fields. Sometimes it seems as if few in positions of power have the strength to resist the temptation of generating vast sums of money via devious if not downright dishonest means.

Whether it be profiting from *manufactured* arms conflicts or manipulating financial markets, history proves greed is often the rule and not the exception when it comes to the global elite's pursuit of wealth – or, perhaps more pertinently and disturbingly, when it comes to their pursuit of greater wealth.

Many argue that when it comes to greed and corruption the medical sector is no different to other lucrative business sectors. This seems a strange accusation given most in the medical field, including doctors, nurses and hospital staffers, embark on their careers out of a compassionate and genuine desire to care for the sick.

Unfortunately, there are powers-that-be whose motives are not so noble. Collectively and unofficially called the *Medical Industrial Complex*, they comprise a surprisingly large number of individuals, corporations, government health services, medical equipment manufacturers and suppliers, and, dare we say it, hangers-on. Those in the latter category include the likes of health systems consultants, insurers, banking executives, accountants, lawyers, construction company reps and even realtors.

However, the so-called *Big Three* in this complex are readily identifiable. They are 'Organized Medicine' (the medical profession as a whole), the Food & Drug Administration (FDA) and, of course, the pharmaceutical industry – let's not forget them.

For readers outside of America, replace *FDA* with your government agency responsible for *allegedly* protecting and promoting public health in your country.

To put the Medical Industrial Complex into perspective, consider this: modern medicine is one of the largest and most profitable industries on the planet. Some medical insiders have described it as America's biggest industry. Not sure it's as big as the *war industry*, but if it ain't, it must be a close second.

At the time of writing, Americans were transfixed, bemused and frustrated by the partisan squabbling surrounding President Obama's attempts to sort out the country's healthcare provisions once and for all.

One who summarizes America's health problems better than most is William A. Collins, a former state representative and former Mayor of Norwalk, Connecticut. In an article dated August 21, 2013, on *OtherWords.org*, Collins says in the US, the health industry's big players focus on making as much money as possible.

Collins claims that those who devise the health system do so with profits in mind, and patients who can't help with that are "shunted off to government services" or snubbed. He's also critical of what he describes as a network of handshakes and private agreements linking hospitals to pharmaceutical company reps and medical equipment manufacturers, claiming this inflates America's health cost as much as the insurance and Big Pharma.

"Fortunately," he says, "the main offenders can be clearly labeled. Chief among them are the health insurers and the drug manufacturers. Big Pharma wields an army of lobbyists and administers large doses of campaign contributions to their friends in Congress".

For those not familiar with the term *Big Pharma*, it's the nickname given to the major pharmaceutical conglomerates which collectively form this multi-trillion dollar industry. Many believe Big Pharma can be compared to the most corrupt banks, media monopolies or oil corporations.

In the pages of this book, we explore the contention that Big Pharma and other participants in the Medical Industrial Complex put profits ahead of patients' wellbeing and dollars ahead of lives.

One of our recurring themes is that all of us must stop giving away complete responsibility to doctors or other medical practitioners. It's time to start looking at these people as they actually are: *advisors* for *you* to make decisions about what's best for *your* body.

Let's face it, most people simply accept whatever pills are prescribed, or surgeries are recommended, or other treatments advised, to them by their doctor without ever questioning. There are hundreds of examples given in this book which prove that approach in dealing with doctors is an unhealthy one (figuratively *and* literally).

The way to avoid becoming another statistic of the Medical Industrial Complex – and more importantly staying healthy or else returning to full health – is to become informed. We assume that might be why you are reading this book: to gain knowledge about modern medicine. And knowledge is the necessary ingredient we all need to make informed decisions about our health.

We have known parents who trusted their doctors who prescribed unnecessary drugs such as *Ritalin* for their children. Unnecessary because these parents later discovered there were other (less aggressive) ways to treat their children's problem. However, at the time they had no idea of the cozy and little-known relationship between doctors and Big Pharma – a relationship they eventually discovered involved financial kickbacks for doctors. Once again, in instances like these, knowledge is power and it has the potential to shield the unwitting against corrupt elements within the Medical Industrial Complex.

An interrelated point we wish to make here is we are definitely not anti-doctors.

Only a fool would deny doctors save lives. When it's a medical emergency and you are in a life-and-death situation, a doctor is *always* your best friend.

However, when you simply have a health problem, or suspected problem, that you wish to resolve or clarify, that's when doctors can sometimes do you a disservice. The disservice we refer to is committing what can only be described as a *medical sin* – such as overprescribing drugs or advising surgery before exploring other less risky treatments.

Such a disservice is usually inadvertent (aka *unintentional* or *careless*), but the end result is the same: *you* suffer the consequences.

Our purpose in writing this book is not to alarm, even though some of the despicable acts committed by medical professionals exposed in the coming pages are indeed alarming. Rather, our intention is to arm readers with "underground knowledge" about the medical system, the major players in that system and their many associates. Once you are aware of certain nefarious trends in modern healthcare, you will be able to spot those trends a mile off and thereby protect yourself and your loves ones from harm, or from being inconvenienced at the very least.

As well as exposing corruption, we wish to enlighten those readers who are not already aware that there are long-standing and rather convincing claims of alternative remedies for so-called *incurable illnesses*. These professed cures, it seems, are either being withheld or blocked by multinational drug companies and/or rigid medical academia. Having researched alternative treatments, we are convinced at least some of these really do cure so-called incurable illnesses, but are being suppressed from the public as they are unpatentable (aka *unprofitable*).

Keep in mind most illnesses and diseases labeled *incurable* are usually only described as such within mainstream medicine in the West. When you consider the number and variety of medical and alternative health treatments and systems available around the world – including traditional Chinese (TCM) and Indian (Ayurveda) and numerous others – "incurable" is possibly a state of mind, or a misnomer even, and there is in all likelihood an existing cure for every known medical ailment. A cure awaiting *discovery* by Western medical professionals.

No matter what your state of health is now – even if you are poorly or, heaven forbid, extremely ill – you *can* build and improve your health. Remember, where there's life there is always hope…so never give up!

Lastly, we must point out we are not doctors or medical professionals, and nothing we, the authors, say in this book should be construed as imparting medical or health advice.

You will note many of the statements throughout are not ours. Rather, they are quotes made in the public domain by medical professionals and others far better qualified than us. (The *others* we refer to include respected authors, medical and health reporters, insiders in various professions and, last but not least, medical watchdogs). Often, but not always, their views on health reflect ours. In every case, we hope, their comments help to give you a better understanding of the medical establishment.

James Morcan & Lance Morcan

CHAPTER 1

The sickness industry

"Big Pharma needs sick people to prosper. Patients, not healthy people, are their customers. If everybody was cured of a particular illness or disease, pharmaceutical companies would lose 100% of their profits on the products they sell for that ailment. What all this means is because modern medicine is so heavily intertwined with the financial profits culture, it's a sickness industry more than it is a health industry."

–The Orphan Conspiracies

As you may have already guessed, we are highly critical of the medical system. We are not alone in this of course. The media (mainstream media and online news and social media sites) constantly inundate us all with reports and allegations – some well-founded, some not – regarding the alarming state of the public healthcare system worldwide.

Transparency International, the Berlin-based global coalition against corruption, brought out the highly publicized *Global Corruption Barometer 2013* – to that point the biggest-ever survey tracking worldwide public opinion on corruption. The healthcare sector corruption figures prominently in that survey.

One of the best summaries of the *Global Corruption Barometer* is to be found on the popular blog site *Health Care Renewal*, which observes in an article dated July 10, 2013, that "the results (of the survey) are not pretty for health care and related sectors world wide and in the US. As expected, these results appear to be causing few echoes".

In the same article, *Health Care Renewal* states that healthcare corruption and its presence in developed countries like the US, is a taboo subject.

The article continues, "Globally, respondents perceived it (healthcare corruption) was a major problem. On average, 17% said they or their family members had to pay bribes in connection with medical and healthcare.

"While the US did not have the worst results, our numbers were not very good...More than one-third (43%) of respondents thought that US health care is corrupt...For comparison, the proportions of people who thought the health care sector is corrupt were 24% in Canada, 28% in France, 48% in Germany, 47% in Japan, and 19% in the United Kingdom...Thus, this survey confirmed that health care corruption is a global problem, and that a large proportion of people in the US believe it is a major problem here".

UK peer-reviewed journal *BMC International Health and Human Rights, which estimates healthcare expenditures globally total 3 trillion US dollars,* indicates it's little wonder this sector is vulnerable to corruption. In an article dated May 3, 2012 and published on its respected *biomedcentral.com* website, *BMC* highlights the huge expense associated with the procurement of the many services the sector offers, and points out that the nature of healthcare is such that the demand is not fully predictable and often exceeds supply.

"Health care systems also tend to have weak or non-existent rules and regulations, lack of accountability, information imbalances between providers and patients and suppliers and providers, and low salaries for health care professionals and public officials. These characteristics of the health sector make it susceptible to corruption."

BMC also claims that theft, diversion and resale of drugs are other sources of corruption that occur at the distribution point of the pharmaceutical supply chain. Examples listed include theft without falsification of inventory records, dispensing of drugs to patients who did not actually attend the pharmacy or clinic, recording of drugs as dispensed to legitimate patients but the patients do not receive them, and dispensing of drugs to patients who pay for them but the health care provider keeps the funds.

The article also gives examples of "illegal kickbacks" to surgeons and false claims allegations, stating that, in one case, "Physicians were allegedly awarded vacations, gifts and annual 'consulting fees' as high as $200,000 in return for physician endorsements of their implants or use of them in operations".

BMC states that the medical device industry, especially in orthopaedics, is an area where there are relatively large sums of money involved and thus there is a susceptibility to corruption.

Clearly, healthcare corruption is a global problem – and a major one at that. Certainly, that's the perception of the majority of independent analysts. Most alarming, or at least *as* alarming, is the reluctance – or downright unwillingness – of those involved to discuss the problem.

Now why is this? Is it because guilty parties are afraid that discussion could lead to investigation of corrupt practices? And are those same parties afraid of what an investigation will uncover?

America's public health is in the spotlight big-time following the January 2015 release of Steven Brill's bestselling book, *America's Bitter Pill: Politics, Backroom Deals, and the Fight to Fix Our Broken Healthcare System.*

Billed as a "fly-on-the-wall account of the fight, amid an onslaught of lobbying, to pass a 961-page law aimed at fixing America's largest, most dysfunctional industry—an industry larger than the entire economy of France," *America's Bitter Pill* is described as "a sweeping narrative of how the Affordable Care Act, or Obamacare, was written, how it is being implemented, and, most important, how it is changing—and failing to change—the rampant abuses in the healthcare industry."

Brill, a graduate of Yale Law School, pulls no punches in his dissection of the industry.

The book's splurge reads:

"It's a penetrating chronicle of how the profiteering that Brill first identified in his *Time* cover story continues, despite Obamacare. And it is the first complete, inside account of how President Obama persevered to push through the law, but then failed to deal with the staff incompetence and turf wars that crippled its implementation.

"Brill questions all the participants in the drama, including the president, to find out what happened and why.

"He asks the head of the agency in charge of the Obamacare website how and why it crashed. And he tells the cliffhanger story of the tech wizards who swooped in to rebuild it.

"Brill gets drug lobbyists to open up on the deals they struck to protect their profits in return for supporting the law… Brill is there with patients when they are denied cancer care at a hospital, or charged $77 for a box of gauze pads. Then he asks the multimillion-dollar executives who run the hospitals to explain why.

"He even confronts the chief executive of America's largest health insurance company and asks him to explain an incomprehensible Explanation of Benefits his company sent to Brill. And he's there as a group of young entrepreneurs gamble millions to use Obamacare to start a hip insurance company in New York's Silicon Alley".

These excerpts from the promotional material for *America's Bitter Pill* cover some of the major culprits in the ongoing corruption of the healthcare industry. Namely, these are – Big Pharma, hospital management executives, politicians and insurance companies.

> *"Our primary health care should begin on the farm and in our hearts, and not in some laboratory of the biotech and pharmaceutical companies."*
>
> *–Gary Hopkins, US health professional and author.*

Chief medical officer for the American Cancer Society, oncologist Dr. Otis Brawley, who has publicly labeled US healthcare "a subtle form of corruption," has long been a frontline critic of unnecessary medical procedures and tests in the medical sector – in particular routine prostate cancer screening of men.

Dr. Brawley's thoughts on US healthcare are well aired in an article dated April 24, 2012, written by columnist Susan Perry and published on the Minneapolis community news site *MinnPost.com*. In it, she advises subscribers that, on the subject of prostate cancer screening, Dr. Brawley has pointed out repeatedly that the scientific evidence doesn't support it — and stating that anybody who says otherwise is "not telling the truth."

The article reports on an address Dr. Brawley gave to a group of medical reporters at the annual conference of the Association of Health Care Journalists in Atlanta. An excerpt from the article follows:

"Brawley also talked in his speech about how 'the whole discussion about health care and health-care reform seemed to lack the fact that there were people out there who were suffering. There were people out there dying.' He quoted a saying used by the Marines: 'We are Americans. We leave no one behind.'

"It's a message, Brawley said, that appears to have eluded many of the politicians and others who are developing our health-care policies. 'We are Americans, and we leave a lot of people behind in our health-care system,' he said.

"He also mentioned how pharmaceutical companies are able to make a minor change in a drug that is about to go off patent and then market it as a new – and, of course, much more expensive – drug, even though it's essentially the same medication. His example was AstraZeneca's transformation of the heartburn drug *Prilosec* into *Nexium*.

"Brawley also criticized the medical community for adopting medical treatments long before their benefits – or safety – have been proven."

The *MinnPost.com* article mentioned that Brawley also cited autologous bone marrow transplantation for breast cancer (widely used in the late 1980s and 1990s), despite the fact that nobody had done any studies to prove that it actually worked.

"Who's at fault for this corruption?" the same article asks. "All of us. 'Quite honestly, it's the doctors, it's the hospitals, it's the hospital system, it's the insurers, it's the drug companies, it's the lawyers,' he said.

"What we desperately need to do is not reform health care," said Brawley. "We need to transform how we view health care. We need to become more appreciative of health-care prevention efforts."

We have already established that corruption in the healthcare sector is not limited to the West. It's a worldwide scourge.

If reports coming out of the Indian subcontinent and neighboring countries are accurate, corruption there is especially rife. A front-page article headed 'Bribe for every service,' dated January 16, 2015, in Bangladesh's *Daily Star* newspaper is a case in point. The article claims that corruption and irregularity rule the country's drug administration "where money can buy licences and registrations for low-quality, counterfeit medicines".

The reporter says the Directorate General of Drug Administration's regulatory mechanism is weak, and he refers to a Transparency International Bangladesh study he says reveals "many of its officials and employees join hands with unscrupulous officials of medicine companies to indulge in corruption". He accuses DGDA officials of taking bribes from medicine companies for various services, and says, according to the study, major corruption takes place in issuance and renewal of drug licences as well as handover and change of ownerships.

> *"Pharmaceutical companies always put profit before humans."*
>
> *–Dr. Shaikh Tanveer Ahmed*

Despite the gloom and doom surrounding the Medical Industrial Complex, all is not lost in our opinion. Many good people remain within the healthcare system and devote their lives to improving the quality of their patients' lives.

Possibly a good analogy is corrupt government administrations. If only 1% of politicians are destructive or deceptive in any government, that can undo the good work of an entire administration. Same sometimes applies with the medical system where a few bad eggs at the very top of the medical establishment can undermine an entire industry of otherwise honest and patient-serving professionals.

Modern technology may eventually empower the public and provide a path to a fairer healthcare system.

One subscriber to the technology-as-a-medical-solution theory is Eric Topol, MD, a professor of translational genomics and the director of the Scripps Translational Science Institute in La Jolla, California. Topol, who is described as a pioneer of the medicine of the future, is also author of the bestselling book, *The Patient Will See You Now: The Future of Medicine is in Your Hands.*

The book's splurge reads as follows:

"In this new era, patients will control their data and be emancipated from a paternalistic medical regime in which 'the doctor knows best.' Mobile phones, apps, and attachments will literally put the lab and the ICU in our pockets. Computers will replace physicians for many diagnostic tasks, and enormous data sets will give us new means to attack conditions that have long been incurable. In spite of these benefits, the path forward will be complicated: some in the medical establishment will resist these changes, and digitized medicine will raise serious issues surrounding privacy. Nevertheless, the result – better, cheaper, and more humane health care for all – will be worth it. *The Patient Will See You Now* is essential reading for anyone who thinks they deserve better health care".

It seems readers are resonating with Topol's book if reviewers' comments are anything to go by.

However, perhaps Topol himself should have the final say to round off this chapter. Here's a quote (from his book) that caught our eye: "Increasing frustration and vexing aspects of health care today may influence a bottoms up movement, propelled by smartphones and social networks for improving the future of medicine".

CHAPTER 2

The political impatience that kills patients

"It is amazing that people who think we cannot afford to pay for doctors, hospitals, and medication somehow think that we can afford to pay for doctors, hospitals, medication and a government bureaucracy to administer it."

–Thomas Sowell, American author, social commentator and Francis Boyer Award-winner

In the foreword, you'll recall retired pharmacist Denis Toovey says in a career spanning 40 years he has seen many examples of patients falling through the cracks in the health system as a direct result of health providers focusing on high patient turnover on a 'fee-for-service' basis with no guarantee of results.

As alarming, if not more so, is his observation that "All too often health professionals have to work within systems created by politicians and administrators that allow for zero direct responsibility for patient outcomes."

The role politics and politicians play in a country's health is worthy of scrutiny and is one that has possibly been overlooked by many other independent critiques and critics of the medical establishment.

Denis perhaps sums it up best when he says serious questions need to be asked about a health 'system' in which politicians are often reluctant to invest money in long-term, preventative measures that can take years to show a return on investment.

A politician's future is very much at the whim of voters who are notoriously fickle. Little wonder then that many tend to focus on short-term policies and initiatives instead of long-term ones. Those who don't are very quickly brought into line by their party – be it on the Left or Right of the political spectrum – whose modus operandi, invariably and almost without exception, is to do whatever's needed to win the next election and to stay in power.

That's politics, folks.

In the process, as Denis points out, "short-term tangible things like spending more money to reduce waiting surgical waiting lists (to win votes) instead of dealing with the long term underlying causes" are given priority.

If the wellbeing of constituents, as well as minors and other non-voters – aka *human beings* – wasn't at stake, we'd say this is rather naughty of our elected representatives. As people's health and, indeed, their very lives are at stake, we'd say this practice or policy, call it what you will, is downright deplorable.

When politics is thrown into the medical melting pot and stirred up with those other *essential* ingredients – namely Big Pharma, hospitals, the medical academic establishment, hospital supply and equipment companies, and other key players in the Medical Industrial Complex – the practice can only be described as seriously corrupt.

Making short-term medical policies, in the case of vote-hungry, power-mad politicians, and pandering to those same policies, in the case of greedy elements within the medical establishment, when lives and health are on the line is unforgivable.

How refreshing it would be if the government of the day announced it was replacing its "ambulance at the bottom of the cliff" health policy with a 10 or 15-year, or, better still, a 20-year vision for the country's health. A vision that requires investment in long-term preventative measures and that encourages a holistic approach.

Alas, the nature of politics and politicians is that no such change will likely occur. Equally, the current system – a system in which cures for diseases and other ailments come a distant second to just treating symptoms – suits the big pharmaceutical companies and their kind just fine. So no change can be expected any time soon from that quarter either.

At the end of the day, we, the common people, have two choices: we can force the politicians to listen or, better still, we can take responsibility for our own health. The obvious advantage in the latter choice is that it's actionable immediately and doesn't rely on a change of government and/or a new type of political leader to emerge.

Be warned, taking responsibility for your own health is not without its challenges. It requires research and no small amount of courage. And, as Denis Toovey warns in the foreword, "Some health professionals do not take too kindly to patients who want to be involved in decisions about their treatment."

So, be prepared for some battles with your doctor. We know from personal experience they don't always welcome questions about the (inevitable) side-effects of prescription drugs or suggestions that natural medicine or a health supplement *may* be a better alternative than a 'quick-fix' pill for certain ailments.

> *"The medical profession is unconsciously irritated by lay knowledge."*
>
> *–John Steinbeck, East of Eden*

CHAPTER 3

Do drug companies make drugs or money?

"It is clear from the evidence presented... that the pharmaceutical industry does a biased job of disseminating evidence – to be surprised by this would be absurd – whether it is through advertising, drug reps, ghostwriting, hiding data, bribing people, or running educational programmes for doctors."

–Ben Goldacre, British physician, academic and science writer

Many people are alive today because of prescription drugs, and many more are enjoying a better quality of life because of prescription drugs. Let us be clear and unequivocal about that. And unsubstantiated criticism of the pharmaceutical industry, or any industry for that matter, does no-one any good.

We kept all that front of mind when conducting our research for this book.

Unfortunately, the inescapable fact is that much of the good Big Pharma does is undone by mistakes, dubious business practices, (reported/confirmed cases of) fraud and, quite simply, by greed.

Much has been written about Big Pharma in recent years. One of the most informative books on the industry is *The Truth About Drug Companies*, by Marcia Angell, M.D., former editor of the prestigious *New England Journal of Medicine*.

The book's blurb reads (abridged):

"Currently Americans spend a staggering $200 billion each year on prescription drugs. As Dr. Angell powerfully demonstrates, claims that high drug prices are necessary to fund research and development are unfounded: The truth is that drug companies funnel the bulk of their resources into the marketing of products of dubious benefit. Meanwhile, as profits soar, the companies brazenly use their wealth and power to push their agenda through Congress, the FDA, and academic medical centers.

"Zeroing in on hugely successful drugs like AZT (the first drug to treat HIV/AIDS), Taxol (the best-selling cancer drug in history), and the blockbuster allergy drug Claritin, Dr. Angell demonstrates exactly how new products are brought to market. Drug companies, she shows, routinely rely on publicly funded institutions for their basic research; they rig clinical trials to make their products look better than they are; and they use their legions of lawyers to stretch out government-granted exclusive marketing rights for years. They also flood the market with copycat drugs that cost a lot more than the drugs they mimic but are no more effective.

"*The Truth About the Drug Companies* is a searing indictment of an industry that has spun out of control".

Within the book itself, Dr. Angell describes the unethical and at times inhumane pharmaceutical industry she witnessed in her 21 years spent as the first female editor-in-chief of *The New England Journal of Medicine*. She also gives numerous examples to prove beyond dispute that the world's biggest drug companies have grown so powerful they are now able to pull the strings and call many of the shots in medical academia, health research and even the way doctors and nurses go about their work. Meanwhile, the public, including more and more of the poor, invalid and elderly, are unable to meet the cost of rapidly increasing prescription drug prices.

In a 2014 video interview with the University of Utah Health Sciences-powered *Algorithms for Innovation,* Dr. Angell said the relationship between pharmaceutical companies, governments and medical academia has become far too symbiotic and cozy.

"They (drug companies) get government-granted monopoly rights, patents and exclusive marketing rights. So, they really are doing very well. Society is taking good care of them. It seems to me that society could ask for something in return. And to say, look, as a price of some of these goodies that we give you, you cannot stop making antibiotics or vaccines or important drugs. This is a part of what you have to do to be so richly rewarded in our society."

"We actually have some shortages in important and even life-saving drugs," Dr. Angell went on to state in the Algorithms for Innovation interview. "And why is that? Because the drug companies don't find them particularly profitable."

The obvious implication in Dr. Angell's expert assessment is that Big Pharma is no longer fixated on creating and manufacturing revolutionary drugs, but has instead become more focused on marketing existing products and maintaining control over the marketplace in order to continue to expand its vast fortunes.

Perhaps scarier still, Dr. Angell, who is currently Senior Lecturer in the Department of Social Medicine at Harvard Medical School, spoke in the same interview of the subservience academic medicine has toward the pharmaceutical industry. Subservience she suggested is mostly due to the fact that Big Pharma finances (either directly or indirectly) more and more research on drugs – especially their own products. For example, drug companies pay medical schools vast sums of money for royalties on their discoveries related to new drugs.

During her tenure overseeing the content of *The New England Journal of Medicine*, Dr. Angell said she eventually realized Big Pharma "were buying the hearts and minds of faculties and medical schools."

Of course, Big Pharma would not have the ability to covertly pull the strings of so many interrelated facets of the medical establishment were it not for their financial empires.

For an insight into the profitability of the major pharmaceutical companies, take a gander at the top performers on the latest *Fortune 500* list. (*Fortune 500* being *Fortune Magazine's* annual list of the top 500 US companies – publicly and privately listed – according to their gross revenues).

At the time of writing, the *2014 Fortune 500 list* was the latest available. One of the best summaries of the pharmaceutical companies (drug wholesalers, chain pharmacies, pharmacy benefit managers (PBMs), and pharmaceutical manufacturers) we could find is on the very professional *DrugChannels.net* site. Compiled by Dr. Adam J. Fein, CEO of Drug Channels Institute, it's an eye-opener for the uninformed.

As Dr. Fein informs the public, his data "will help you 'follow the dollar' and understand how drug channel intermediaries make money."

The good doctor compares the fortunes of the eight listed drug channels companies (AmerisourceBergen, Cardinal Health, CVS Caremark, Express Scripts, McKesson, Omnicare, Rite Aid, and Walgreens) with *Fortune 500's* 12 pharmaceutical manufacturers and a separate survey of independent pharmacies.

Dr. Fein reports "The 2013, median revenues for the eight drug channel companies were $95.1 billion, up 1.4% vs. 2012. Median revenues for the manufacturer group were $17.5 billion… The revenues of the 12 largest pharmaceutical manufacturers on the Fortune 500 list range from $67.2 billion (Pfizer) to $5.5 billion (Celgene)".

In the report he quotes 2012 data supplied by the National Community Pharmacists Association's 2013 *NCPA Digest*, which shows that independent pharmacies had higher profitability than the eight largest drug channels companies, including PBMs.

Dr. Fein also observes that, "In 2013…investment returns reflected last year's strong stock market performance".

The median Total Return to Investors in 2013 as reported from *Fortune's* list is detailed as follows: 8 Drug Channels companies: +65.8% (range: +30.1% to +272.1%); 12 Drug Manufacturers: +34.8% (range: +7.3% to +115.3%).

Starting to get the picture? Big Pharma is mighty profitable and becoming more so each and every year.

So what's the main modus operandi of these mighty profitable pharmaceutical companies? *The New York Times* kinda asks this same question in an article (dated June 2, 2014) headed 'Do Drug Companies Make Drugs or Money?'

New York Times' contributor Andrew Ross Sorkin quotes one Mike Pearson, chief executive of Valeant Pharmaceuticals International, whom he claims was "waxing poetic last week about the virtues of his company. He was doing so as he was trying to sell shareholders of Allergan, the maker of *Botox*, on his company's $53 billion takeover bid".

Sorkin continues, "Here's what the investment firm Sterne Agee said in its recent research report: 'The Allergan executive team is one of the best and most shareholder-focused in the pharmaceutical industry.' The numbers tell the story: Allergan's stock is up 290 percent over the last five years.

"And so what we're left with isn't a tale about a brilliantly innovative drug company trying to buy a mismanaged fixer-upper; it's quite the opposite. Valeant, desperate for ways to increase its revenue, needs a cash cow to milk until it can find the next one".

According to Forbes contributor John LaMattina, in an item (dated July 29, 2014) on *Forbes.com*, the title of Sorkin's *New York Times* article "was taken from Harvard professor, Bill George, who asked: 'Is the role of leading large pharmaceutical companies to discover lifesaving drugs or to make money for shareholders through financial engineering?' "

Good question!

LaMattina, who reports on developments in the pharmaceutical industry, says Professor George's question was prompted by the spate of companies seeking to merge with foreign companies with the ultimate intent of lowering their corporate tax rates.

"However," LaMattina asserts, "these comments play on the public's concern that the pharmaceutical industry is primarily focused on making money – not drugs. This reinforces the notion that companies focus only on profits, and preferentially work on life-style enhancing drugs, or drugs that offer minimum improvements over existing therapies but for which companies charge exorbitant prices.

"The problem is that running a biopharmaceutical company is an expensive and high risk endeavor. If you cannot generate a very significant profit, you can't survive".

LaMattina concludes, "As crass as it may sound, the companies responsible for discovering and developing the next medical breakthroughs have to do so in a way that generates significant profits. If they don't do that, investors will turn to other places to invest their money, and the companies will shrivel up and either be sold to another company or die.

"So the answer to the Sorkin/George question is 'both'. A pharma company's business is making drugs – and, in doing so it had better make profits".

No-one can object to the drug companies making profits. Surely that's the aim of all companies – to make profits.

But how much is too much?

CHAPTER 4

So how much is too much?

Our criticism of Big Pharma is tempered by the knowledge that – as we acknowledge more than once elsewhere in this book – products developed, manufactured and marketed by the pharmaceutical companies save lives. (Some would argue they cost lives, too, but that's another story).

However, we keep coming back to the questions that crop up whenever the pharmaceutical companies and their modus operandi are analyzed. Questions like: Why is so little money ploughed back into research? Why the continuing emphasis on treatments ahead of cures? And, regarding revenues and profits, how much is too much?

BBC News addresses this very issue in a report aired on November 6, 2014 under the title 'Pharmaceutical industry gets high on fat profits.' The report asks people to imagine an industry that generates higher profit margins than any other and is no stranger to multi-billion dollar fines for malpractice.

"Throw in widespread accusations of collusion and over-charging, and banking no doubt springs to mind. In fact, the industry described above is responsible for the development of medicines to save lives and alleviate suffering, not the generation of profit for its own sake".

The *BBC News* report reminds us that pharmaceutical companies have, by far, developed most medicines known to Man, but have profited big-time in the process – "and not always by legitimate means".

It continues, "Last year, US giant Pfizer, the world's largest drug company by pharmaceutical revenue, made an eye-watering 42% profit margin… five pharmaceutical companies made a profit margin of 20% or more…With some drugs costing upwards of $100,000 for a full course, and with the cost of manufacturing just a tiny fraction of this, it's not hard to see why…

"Drug companies justify the high prices they charge by arguing that their research and development (R&D) costs are huge. On average, only three in 10 drugs launched are profitable, with one of those going on to be a blockbuster with $1bn-plus revenues a year…

"But … drug companies spend far more on marketing drugs – in some cases twice as much – than on developing them. And besides, profit margins take into account R&D costs".

The report concludes that the industry also argues that the wider value of the drug needs to be considered. However, it (*BBC News*) rightly points out that just because you can charge a high price for something does not necessarily mean you should. Especially when you factor in the lives at stake in the healthcare field.

The problem with that is – as we see it – the pharmaceutical companies and the shareholders they answer to would quickly dismiss such a rationale. They're solely focused on the bottom line: profit.

Profit is not necessarily a dirty word when it comes to healthcare. We happen to believe capitalism, if managed properly, can actually work well in medicine. Profit incentives can spark imaginations in pharmacists and healthcare entrepreneurs and doctors as there's the reward aspect in capitalism which motivates people to find medical cures.

Otherwise, as evidenced in the past in places like Eastern Europe, when things go to the other extreme and there's too much government interference it can be just as crippling and corrupting for essential services such as healthcare. With little to no financial rewards on offer under communism, or even under some forms of socialism, most workers are less motivated – medical and healthcare workers included.

Somehow there needs to be a balance between governments and non-profit review committees to ensure mainstream medicine has a social conscience whilst still allowing the free market to work its magic.

Criticism of pharmaceutical companies has been taken a step further by internal medicine specialist-turned author Professor Peter C. Gøtzsche whose hard-hitting book *Deadly Medicines and Organised Crime: How Big*

Pharma Has Corrupted Healthcare basically equates the drug companies to organized crime.

The book's introduction states that Gøtzsche exposes the pharmaceutical industries and their charade of fraudulent behavior, both in research and marketing where the morally repugnant disregard for human lives is the norm. "He convincingly draws close comparisons with the tobacco conglomerates, revealing the extraordinary truth behind efforts to confuse and distract the public and their politicians.

"The book addresses, in evidence-based detail, an extraordinary system failure caused by widespread crime, corruption, bribery and impotent drug regulation in need of radical reforms".

Professor Gøtzsche himself states the main reason we take so many drugs is that drug companies don't sell drugs, they sell lies about drugs. "This is what makes drugs so different from anything else in life... Virtually everything we know about drugs is what the companies have chosen to tell us and our doctors... the reason patients trust their medicine is that they extrapolate the trust they have in their doctors into the medicines they prescribe. The patients don't realize that, although their doctors may know a lot about diseases and human physiology and psychology, they know very, very little about drugs that hasn't been carefully concocted and dressed up by the drug industry".

Professor Gøtzsche, incidentally, graduated as a Master of Science in biology and chemistry in 1974 and as a physician in 1984 – so he's well qualified to speak out on such matters. A Danish physician turned medical researcher, he worked with clinical trials and regulatory affairs in the drug industry from 1975 to 1983, and at hospitals in Copenhagen from 1984 to 1995.

The professor continues, "If you don't think the system is out of control, please email me and explain why drugs are the third leading cause of death... If such a hugely lethal epidemic had been caused by a new bacterium or a virus, or even one-hundredth of it, we would have done everything we could to get it under control".

In the pharmaceutical industry's haste to get drugs to market, critics say safety usually comes a distance second to profits. Little wonder then that mistakes occur and the line between legitimate and spurious business practices is oftentimes blurred.

We explore this untenable situation in the next chapter.

CHAPTER 5

Dangerous drugs Big Pharma doesn't want you to know about

*"So, if we're to make any sense of the mess that the
pharmaceutical industry – and my profession – has made
of the academic literature, then we need an amnesty: we
need a full and clear declaration of all the distortions, on
missing data, ghostwriting, and all the other
activity... to prevent the ongoing harm that they still
cause."*

–Ben Goldacre, British physician, academic and science writer

Sadly, the path the drug companies have followed, and continue to follow, is a long, rocky one littered with mistakes – mistakes that have been fatal for some; mistakes Big Pharma's critics have labeled criminal; mistakes some claim are all too often more deliberate than accidental and therefore can hardly be referred to as *mistakes*.

Certainly the history of court cases involving Big Pharma is equally long and rocky with fines against the industry's major players totaling many, many billions of dollars.

Our research has turned up numerous case studies that highlight just how "mistake-prone" this industry is and how often drug companies have ended up on the wrong side of the law. We include just a few of these in this chapter.

The first headline worth repeating was this one on the front page of the *Daily Mail's* edition of July 2, 2012: 'GlaxoSmithKline to pay $3billion fine after pleading guilty to healthcare fraud – the biggest in U.S. History.'

The report reads in part: "GlaxoSmithKline paid U.S. medics to prescribe potentially dangerous medicines to adults and children. It handed out cash as well as everything from Madonna concert tickets to pheasant-hunting trips. Authorities branded GSK as 'cheaters who thought they could make an easy profit at the expense of public safety, taxpayers, and millions of Americans.'

"The enormous settlement – believed to be the largest ever for a drugs firm – covers offences relating to some of GSK's best-selling drugs between 1997 and 2004.

"It bribed doctors to prescribe Paxil to children even though the authorities had not approved its use for under-18s. The controversial depression drug has been linked to a higher risk of suicide both in the US and here, where it is known as Seroxat.

"The main charges also relate to Wellbutrin, another drug for treating depression, and Avandia, a diabetes treatment…"

The *Daily Mail* report advises readers that GSK, which is based in West London, is Britain's fifth biggest public company with a market valuation of $113 billion and a roster of household names that includes *Lucozade*, *Aquafresh*, *Ribena* and *Horlicks*. "It accounts for almost 5 per cent of the benchmark FTSE 100 index and is a favourite investment for pension fund managers".

According to the report, GSK agreed to pay a fine of around $1 billion to the US authorities and a further payment of around $2 billion in civil settlements to state and federal authorities.

"The company's marketeers promoted Wellbutrin as a weight loss treatment when it was approved only for treating depression…

"Carmen Ortiz, the US attorney for Massachusetts, said: 'GSK's sales force bribed physicians to prescribe GSK products using every imaginable form of high priced entertainment, from Hawaiian vacations to paying doctors millions of dollars to go on speaking tours, to a European pheasant hunt, to tickets to Madonna concerts'. "

We think that last statement attributed to Carmen Ortiz is interesting as it mirrors our theory that at least some of the blame can be attributed to doctors in our critique of the Medical Industrial Complex.

Many other news stories and independent assessments of medical corruption also match this belief.

For example, on September 2, 2009, *The Guardian* ran this article (abridged) from Andrew Clark in New York:

"Pfizer, the world's largest drugs company, has been hit with the biggest criminal fine in US history as part of a $2.3bn settlement with federal prosecutors for mispromoting medicines and for paying kickbacks to compliant doctors.

"In a blow to its reputation in the eyes of doctors and patients, Pfizer pleaded guilty to misbranding the painkiller Bextra, withdrawn from the market in 2004, by promoting the drug for uses that were not approved by medical regulators."

The NY-based pharmaceutical company also settled civil allegations regarding under-the-table payments to doctors who prescribed other drug products – even though the company itself has continued to deny this ever occurred at the time of writing.

The Guardian article continues, "Under an out-of-court deal with the US department of justice, a Pfizer subsidiary, Pharmacia & Upjohn, is paying a criminal fine of $1.3bn (nearly £800m), a record in American judicial history. Pfizer is also paying $1bn in civil settlements to Medicare, Medicaid and other government health insurance schemes to reimburse improper prescriptions.

"Prosecutors said the payments reflected the 'size and seriousness' of Pfizer's infringements. Tom Perrelli, the associate attorney general, said it was a victory for the public over 'those who seek to earn a profit through fraud'.

"Perrelli said: 'Every year we lose tens of billions of dollars in Medicare and Medicaid funds to fraud. Those billions represent healthcare dollars that could be spent on medicine, elder care or emergency room visits but instead are spent on medicines or devices that are simply not effective for patients to whom they are prescribed'."

Unfortunately, none of these fraudulent activities conducted by drug companies are isolated incidents or particularly out-of-the-norm.

On December 26, 2013, under the heading 'Ethics: End of the hard sell?,' the *Financial Times* reported on a $2.2billion fine pharmaceutical giant Johnson and Johnson was slugged with for promoting drugs not approved as safe.

The article states, "When Johnson & Johnson wanted to boost prescriptions of Natrecor, a heart medicine, it channeled more than $100,000 through a subsidiary company to a sympathetic nurse. In exchange, she spoke favourably about the drug in talks, trained colleagues on how to use it, and put her name on an article in a medical journal to boost sales.

"This ruse, part of an aggressive marketing campaign, was not carried out in the developing world but the US, where J&J paid a $2.2bn fine last month for practices stretching back over a decade. It was only the latest in an escalating series of penalties against the pharmaceutical industry for the way it markets its products.

"Western drug groups have rapidly expanded their sales – and sales tactics – in emerging markets over the past 10 years. Now regulatory scrutiny is catching up, not just in the US but around the world, including in China, where GlaxoSmithKline has been accused of paying up to $500m in bribes to local doctors."

The *Financial Times* report continues, "In the US alone, cumulative fines from whistleblower and government prosecutions against the industry reached $20bn in the period 1991-2010, suggesting something is wrong with the system. In less than three years since then, companies have been hit with further penalties totalling more than $13bn.

"Last year, Eli Lilly paid $29m to the US Securities and Exchange Commission after evidence showed it offered discounts to fund bribes to win business in Brazil and Kazakhstan. Pfizer was fined $60m for activities including "incentive trips" to Greece for Bulgarian doctors who agreed to meet prescription targets for its drugs".

Our filed list of case studies goes on...and on...and on. It's a depressingly long list. There's the $1.5bn Xxxxxx (2012) case concerning the illegal promotion of the antipsychotic drug Xxxxxxxx. (*Names redacted for legal reasons*). There's also the $1.42bn Xxx Xxx (2009) case for wrongly promoting the antipsychotic drug Xxxxxxx; there's the $950m Xxxxx (2011) case over illegally promoting painkiller Xxxxx.

Some quick research online will reveal the redacted names (above) of the drugs and drug companies involved.

Need we go on? Okay, we don't want to depress you any further...

However, it would be remiss of us not to refer you to *FoodMatters.tv*, an excellent wellness site we stumbled across. Under the heading '15 Most Dangerous Drugs Big Pharma Don't Want You to Know About,' it lists exactly that – the 15 most dangerous etc. etc.

FoodMatters' correspondent says, "Drugs are so plagued with safety problems, it is a wonder they're on the market at all" and "it's a testament to Big Pharma's greed and our poor regulatory processes that they are".

The correspondent labels the following drugs "dangerous": *Lipitor* and *Crestor, Yaz* and *Yasmin, Lyrica, Topomax* and *Lamictal, Humira, Prolia* and *TNF Blockers, Chantix, Ambien, Tamoxifen, Boniva, Prempro* and *Premarin.*

FoodMatters provides an explanation for its opposition to each of the above-named drugs.

For example, in the case of *Lipitor*, the correspondent asks, "Why is Lipitor the bestselling drug in the world? Because every adult with high LDL (low-density lipoprotein) or fear of high LDL is on it. (And also 2.8 million children, says *Consumer Reports*.) No one is going to say statins don't prevent heart attack in high-risk patients (though diet and exercise have worked in high-risk groups too). But doctors will say statins are so over-prescribed that more patients get their side effects – weakness, dizziness, pain and arthritis – than heart attack prevention. Worse, they think it's old age".

And in the case of *Crestor*, the correspondent says, "Crestor is so highly linked to rhabdomyolysis it is doubly criticised: Public Citizen calls it a Do Not Use and **the FDA's David Graham named it one of the five most dangerous drugs before Congress**".

So, next time your doctor writes out a prescription, or your local pharmacist hands a prescription to you, or you pop a pill the TV ads insist is "safe" keep all the above in mind. Certainly there are some *miracle drugs* and even, dare we admit it, some *cures* out there in *Big Pharma Country*, but equally there's some highly dubious and downright dangerous drugs – and we're not just talking about the illegal or illicit variety!

CHAPTER 6

Vaccinating children – Is it the smart thing for parents to do?

"I got dragged into the vaccine issue kicking and screaming because I was going around the country suing coal-burning power plants and talking about the dangers of mercury coming from those plants, and almost everywhere I stopped or I spoke there were women there—very eloquent, articulate, grounded people—who said, 'You have to look at the biggest factor of mercury in American children now, and it's vaccines, and we need you to look at the science. And I resisted for a long time but I started reading the science after a while ... I've brought hundreds and hundreds of successful lawsuits, and most of them have involved scientific controversies. I'm comfortable reading science and dissecting it, and discerning the difference between junk science and real science. When I started looking at it, what I saw was very alarming, which is we were giving huge amounts of mercury to our children. A lot of it has been taken out of vaccines, but there's still an extraordinary amount in vaccines—in particular the flu vaccine."

–Robert F. Kennedy Jr. in April 2015 on *Real Time with Bill Maher.*

Given all the examples listed in previous chapters of drug companies' fraudulent activities, can society trust Big Pharma enough to be sure child immunizations are not dangerous?

Is there any limit to the lengths drug companies will go to in order to maximize revenue? And if adult lives aren't safe in this mad pursuit of profits, can we be certain children's lives won't be viewed as expendable as well?

But surely they wouldn't suppress scientific evidence of vaccine dangers when it comes to children? you may ask. *Surely they wouldn't go that far? Right?*

Well, you may be right, but let's break things down a little before reaching any conclusions.

Firstly, it's an indisputable fact that immunizations protect many millions of children every year from potentially deadly diseases, and they save countless lives. It is undeniable that vaccines have all but eradicated a whole host of serious diseases including diphtheria, rubella and smallpox. Polio was also on that list although, alarmingly, it has reportedly been making a comeback in recent years.

Given the apparent overwhelming scientific evidence proving the effectiveness of child immunizations, in legal parlance this seems like it should be *case closed.* However, not all parents, and more significantly not all health industry professionals, agree it's as simple an issue as that. Indeed, some doctors, nurses and other health professionals argue the underreported risks of vaccinating infants far outweigh the protection they provide against certain diseases.

At the time of writing, Californian politicians were considering passing a new law – Senate Bill 277 (SB 277) – making it mandatory for Californian residents to vaccinate their children. As you can imagine, this hasn't gone down well with everyone.

Taking away parents' ability to choose has stirred up the vaccine debate once more – especially in alternative media.

On April 23, 2015, the healthy living website *Elephant* ran an article by health campaigner Elliot Freed, commenting on the issues at stake. In it, Freed hints at complexities that go beyond whether vaccines are safe and effective, stating, "In 1986 vaccine manufacturers were given financial immunity from the damages of their products by congress".

It turns out that law change led to a program that's funded by a 75 cent levy on every vaccine sold.

The article heavily implies that through this legal and/or political loophole, drug companies can repeatedly dodge most claims which attempt to establish a link between vaccines and injury to children.

The *Elephant* article also mentions how more child vaccines than ever contain disease-producing pathogens – more so since liability was eliminated for drug companies producing vaccines. The list of vaccines containing pathogens, according to the article, includes "the MMR, the dTap and the oral polio vaccine".

Because of the financial immunity in the production of vaccines, pharmaceutical manufacturers are now much more focused on developing vaccines than drugs. Easy to understand why: it's a lower risk activity.

Freed continues, "Drugs go through a more rigorous testing process. They are then optional for consumers and consumers and governments can sue pharmaceutical companies for damages caused by the drugs. Vaccines are subject to a less rigorous testing process, saving millions of dollars for each drug sold as a vaccine."

And of course, vaccines need far less advertising costs – especially when governments make their usage mandatory.

"This is not about vaccines for diseases like polio or measles," Freed says. He goes on to predict that many other future vaccines will become mandatory as well. "Where are the infectious epidemics that are killing our children? I don't see them".

If the bill (SB 277) passes, according to Freed, "No state legislator, no school administrator, no doctor and no parent will be able to say no to any chemical mandated by the federal government to be injected into children, so long as it is packaged as a 'vaccine'".

Is this paranoia? Unfounded speculation? A theory only tinfoil hat-wearing conspiracy theorists would believe?

Not according to RFK's son, Robert F. Kennedy, Jr., who has warned the public that a medically induced 'holocaust' is now upon us.

In an article that appeared on *Natural News* on April 26, 2015, the attorney, radio host, environmental activist and author was reported as adding his voice to those against the proposed senate bill.

The article states, "At a recent screening of the powerful new documentary film *Trace Amounts*, which exposes the scientific connection between autism and mercury in vaccines and autism, Robert F. Kennedy, Jr. warned an audience of supportive viewers that vaccines are essentially poison vials causing a 'holocaust' in our country.

"The nephew of former U.S. president John F. Kennedy, RFK Jr. attended the screening in solidarity with Californian parents who are fighting to stop Senate Bill 277 from eliminating their freedom as Californians to exempt their children from 'mandatory' vaccinations. Speaking to the crowd, Kennedy emphasized the proven dangers of vaccines".

" 'They can put anything they want in that vaccine and they have no accountability for it,' stated Kennedy about the vaccine industry, which ironically maintains its own exclusive and unconstitutional exemption from legal liability for vaccines that injure and kill children".

At the April 2015 screening of *Trace Amounts* in California, where not a single invited politician showed up, RFK Jr. received standing ovations as he mentioned how the film helped persuade lawmakers in Oregon to scrap a bill similar to California's SB 277.

Trace Amounts chronicles the true story of Eric Gladen's horrific struggles with mercury poisoning he believes resulted from a thimerosal-loaded tetanus shot. His discoveries led him on a quest for the scientific truth about the potential role of mercury poisoning in the world's current autism epidemic.

The *Natural News* article also mentions that Kennedy "empathized with parents of vaccine-injured children who often have no support from the legal system, and sometimes even from their friends and family members, in addressing the damage caused by vaccine quackery".

It quotes Kennedy as saying, "They get the shot, that night they have a fever of a hundred and three, they go to sleep, and three months later their brain is gone." Lamenting about how vaccine injuries progress, Kennedy adds, "This is a holocaust, what this is doing to our country."

It's worth noting that not all who are opposed to the vaccine law reforms being considered in California, the US and elsewhere in the world are against child immunizations.

Some (anti) campaigners have either had their own children vaccinated or have advised other parents to vaccinate, but also argue that making immunizations mandatory is unconstitutional and against citizens' medical freedom.

Are those who do not vaccinate their own children putting other children, and society as a whole, at risk?

We cannot confidently answer that. Nor, it appears, can anyone. Not with any degree of certainty.

Added to the difficulty of sourcing accurate research and reliable statistics is the problem of widespread corruption highlighted in earlier chapters. Sad but unsurprising in any industry as profitable as Big Pharma.

A February 15, 2015 article about vaccines, published on the *Collective Evolution* website and written by Arjun Walia, nicely summarizes a global trend. Headlined 'The Top 6 Reasons Why Parents Are Choosing Not To Vaccinate Their Kids', the article quotes Walia as saying, "More and more parents around the globe are choosing to opt out of vaccinating themselves and their children".

The article continues, "As a result of this trend that's been gaining more and more momentum, a harsh response has come from the 'pro-vaccine' community-criticizing parents for their decision to not vaccinate. At the end of the day it's not really about 'pro-vaccination' or 'anti-vaccination,' it's not one 'against' the other or about pointing fingers and judgement, it's simply about looking at all of the information from a neutral standpoint. It's about asking questions and communicating so people can make the best possible decisions for themselves and their children.

"Parents love their kids and the vaccine 'controversy' has made it difficult for many parents to know what to do".

Walia says, "Parents who are choosing not to vaccinate their children are not just doing it based on belief, they are doing it based on science and information. This science and information is nowhere near emphasized to the point where the science and information on the other side of the coin is ('pro vaccine').

"Parents who choose not to vaccinate themselves or their children are clearly intelligent, and they should not be made to look like fools. On the other hand, parents who are choosing to vaccinate their children are also intelligent.

"Those who choose to vaccinate should not be made out to be the ones who have made the 'right' decision when there is evidence on both sides of the coin that clearly shows parents who are not vaccinating their children could also be making the 'right' decision".

The article lists (as follows) the top six reasons parents choose not to vaccinate their kids:

1. The Vaccine/Autism Controversy

2. Scientific/Industry Fraud

3. The National Childhood Vaccine Injury Act

4. The Ineffectiveness Of Some Vaccines And Vaccine Injury

5. Vaccine Ingredients

6. Vaccine Safety Evidence Is Not Rock Solid. One Size Does Not Fit All.

In his conclusion, Walia presents a fairly balanced argument that suggests it's time to open up the debate as currently the pro-vaccination lobby is the only one that's being given airtime in the mainstream media.

Besides the fact that pharmaceutical companies cannot be trusted, the other aspect in the equation is that virtually all vaccines are loaded with chemicals and other poisons.

Here's a rundown on some of the damaging ingredients in vaccines on the market today, as listed on the *Healthy Home Economist* website in a 2015 article:

"MSG, antifreeze, phenol (used as a disinfectant), formaldehyde (cancer causing and used to embalm), aluminum (associated with alzheimer's disease and seizures), glycerin (toxic to the kidney, liver, can cause lung damage, gastrointestinal damage and death), lead, cadmium, sulfates, yeast proteins, antibiotics, acetone (used in nail polish remover), neomycin and streptomycin. And the ingredient making the press is thimerosol (more toxic than mercury, a preservative still used in many vaccines, not easily eliminated, can cause severe neurological damage as well as other life threatening autoimmune disease). These vaccines are grown and strained through animal or human tissue, like monkey and dog kidney tissue, chick embryo, calf serum, human diploid cells (the dissected organs of aborted fetuses), pig blood, horse blood and rabbit brain."

The article also states that other countries are waking up to the dangers of vaccines. "In 1975, Japan raised its minimum vaccination age to two years. The country's infant mortality subsequently plummeted to such low levels that Japan now enjoys one of the lowest levels in the Western world

(#3 at last look). In comparison, the United States' infant mortality rate is #33.

(It should be mentioned the Japanese ruling has since been amended. According to the *Vaccination Liberation-Information* site, Japan's health authorities now recommend six vaccinations via injection in the first year of life, and three more in the second year. That, according to the same source, compares to 20 vaccinations in the first two years of life of most American children).

The *Healthy Home Economist* article continues, "In Australia, the flu vaccine was recently suspended (April 2010) for children under 5 because an alarming number of children were showing up in the emergency rooms with febrile convulsions or other vaccine reactions within hours of getting this shot".

After researching the pros and cons of immunizations, and listening to all sides of the debate, we still have NO IDEA what the best decision is for parents to make regarding that most tricky of questions – *to vaccinate or not to vaccinate.*

However, we do agree there needs to be a wider public debate as this issue ain't necessarily as cut and dried as Big Pharma and others in the Medical Industrial Complex would have us believe.

As with many cases involving extreme or polarizing points of view, we suspect the truth regarding child immunizations is probably somewhere in the middle ground. We also disregard (and recommend you do, too) the "evil mega conspiracy" implications some anti-vaccine campaigners trot out just as we disregard the "science is already 100% proven and safe" claims the pro-vaccine lobby loudly trumpets.

We also think that, at the very least, those adults who are happy to vaccinate their children should be demanding en masse that pharmaceutical companies remove all the toxic chemicals and other poisons that are loaded in these vaccines. When you scan the ingredients, which read like they belong in a can of household paint, it's obvious these things just cannot be good for the health and wellbeing of a child's brain or body!

For all we know it may be better for a child to be subjected to all these doses of chemicals and poisons than risk contracting serious diseases like polio, but does that make it right? And is everything that can be done, being done, to make vaccines' ingredients less toxic and safer?

It's unfortunate that only a small percentage of the public are aware of what exactly is in vaccines. If more people were made aware, and if enough demanded less poisonous vaccines, then Big Pharma would be forced to change.

Boycotting products and putting public pressure on corporations and governments can be a very effective way to enforce change. Ultimately, the power rests with the people – *the 99 percent.*

If enough demand change, it will happen. And it does seem at least some changes *are* needed in this most vexing of issues – the vaccination of our children.

CHAPTER 7

Overprescribing blood pressure pills and antidepressants

Is it our imagination or are the goalposts for high blood pressure (BP) ever changing?

It doesn't seem that long ago the "safe" systolic blood pressure (SBP) reading was *your age + 100*. So, for a 60-year-old, your SBP could be 160 over, say, 90 DBP (diastolic blood pressure) without your doctor suddenly becoming flustered and informing you a heart attack or stroke is imminent and immediately prescribing a lifetime course of BP medication.

Then the BP safety guideline dropped to 140 over 90. Imagine how many additional patients that little adjustment resulted in for doctors and medical centers. And perhaps more to the point, imagine how much in additional profits that yielded for the corner pharmacies and the big pharmaceutical companies.

Now all of a sudden – or since 2014 at least – the American Medical Association recommends drugs should be used to treat anyone aged 60 or over whose BP is 150/90 or higher.

That tidbit was gleaned from a February 5, 2014 article in *JAMA*, the *Journal of the AMA*. In that article, *JAMA* states the BP recommendation "is based on evidence statements…in which there is moderate- to high-quality evidence…that in the general population aged 60 years or older, treating high BP to a goal of lower than 150/90 mm Hg reduces stroke, heart failure, and coronary heart disease".

Okay, so that's a reversal of the downward trend we referred to, but it certainly fits the 'moving goalposts' analogy.

That said, we note the American Heart Association (AHA) recommends that BP for an adult aged 20 years or over "should normally be less than 120/80" and if your reading is 140/90 or higher "your doctor will likely want you to begin a treatment program". That's according to AHA's *heart.org* website.

By its reckoning, about one in three American adults has high blood pressure. Little wonder given its BP parameters.

Here in New Zealand, our homeland, the Heart Foundation's BP guideline for healthy adults, according to its website at *heartfoundation.org.nz*, should be below 140/85.

Back to the American Medical Association's take on blood pressure – commenting on AMA's new guidelines, *WebMD*, which promotes itself as "America's healthy living magazine," confirms on its website the AMA guideline sets a higher bar for treatment than the current guideline of 140/90.

WebMD quotes guidelines author Dr. Paul James as saying the recommendations are based on clinical evidence showing that stricter guidelines provided *no additional benefit* to patients. "We really couldn't see additional health benefits by driving blood pressure lower than 150 in people over 60 (years of age)…It was very clear that 150 was the best number".

We wonder how that went down with the drug companies? Not too well, we suspect. The 10-point upward adjustment of the SBP reading is no doubt costing them millions. Or should that read *billions*?

Certainly, the revised BP guidelines didn't go down too well, according to *WebMD*, which reports the AHA expressed reservations. It quotes AHA president-elect Dr. Elliott Antman as saying the AHA is concerned that relaxing the recommendations may expose more persons to the problem of inadequately controlled BP.

Apparently, the AHA's concerns aren't shared by American local government and social issues reporter Aaron Kase who is highly critical of what he describes as the over-prescription of blood pressure meds.

Kase came to our attention courtesy of the American law site *Lawyers.com*, which ran an article first posted in *Medical Malpractice* on August 27, 2012. In that article, Kase (the author) states that, according to a new study, tens of millions of people taking BP medication prescribed by their doctors may be consuming the drugs for no reason.

"The report, which was conducted independently from any drug company money or influence, found the vast majority of people who take meds for hypertension (high blood pressure) see no benefit from them, and do not show reduced levels of heart attack or stroke".

The article continues, "According to the Center for Disease Control, some 1 in 3 adults in America, or 68 million people, have high blood pressure. However, for most of them the condition is considered mild. Historically, even those mild cases are prescribed medication; but the study says the drugs do no good for mild hypertension and could cause harm to patients through side effects".

Kase reports there are dozens of different medications prescribed for high BP, spread across a number of categories – each with its own side effects, ranging from constipation, excessive hair growth, erection problems, rashes and fever to heart palpitations and other adverse reactions.

"A tall price to pay, if the drugs aren't actually helping people live longer," he says.

The writer concludes that, unfortunately, big drugs are big business, and wherever money is involved, motivations can come into question when medications are prescribed to people who might not need them.

Such claims aren't new of course. On January 8, 2012, the UK's *The Observer* reported the BP bar was set at 140/90 whereas 15 years earlier the threshold was 160/100.

And way back in June 2005, *The Seattle Times* reported that, in recent years, expert panels from prestigious medical-research organizations such as the World Health Organization (WHO) and the federal National Institutes of Health (NIH) have called for lower thresholds for blood pressure – and, the report points out, "Behind each of those panels were the giant pharmaceutical companies that manufacture the new and expensive hypertension drugs".

That report concludes, "The drug industry welcomed the new treatment guidelines and marketed them vigorously. Not surprisingly, as doctors followed the new guidelines and treated hypertension at lower readings, sales of the newer drugs increased".

High BP is unquestionably a bigger problem in the West, and many experts attribute that to our higher consumption of salt.

This is touched on in *The Observer* article referred to earlier. It reports that Brazil's Yanomami tribe, whose members eat a diet low in salt and saturated fat and high in fruit, have the lowest mean blood pressure of any population on earth – 95/61.

Nor, apparently, does their blood pressure increase with age. "By contrast, in the west, where people eat an average of 10-12 grams of salt per day, blood pressure rises with age by an average of 0.5mm Hg a year. That may not sound a lot, but over the average lifespan that is a difference of between 35 and 44mm Hg systolic".

The article concludes that the most recent meta-analysis of trials involving more than 6000 people from around the world, found that a reduction in salt intake of just 2 grams a day reduced the risk of cardiovascular events by 20%.

That may well be the case although we suspect that applies to everyday *table salt* and not to pure, unadulterated, unrefined sea salt or Himalayan salt.

Even more depressing than our ever-increasing reliance on drugs to combat high blood pressure is the overprescribing and over-use of antidepressants – especially where children are concerned.

"Suicide rates have not slumped under the onslaught of antidepressants, mood-stabilizers, anxiolytic and anti-psychotic drugs; the jump in suicide rates suggests that the opposite is true. In some cases, suicide risk skyrockets once treatment begins (the patient may feel not only penalized for a justifiable reaction, but permanently stigmatized as malfunctioning). Studies show that self-loathing sharply decreases only in the course of cognitive-behavioral treatment."

–Antonella Gambotto-Burke, The Eclipse: A Memoir of Suicide

Statistically, there's a very good chance you know someone who is taking *Prozac* or some other antidepressant right now. It may be a neighbor, or colleague, or a friend or family member, or, it may be you.

This no doubt has something to do with the readiness of people to talk about their depression or even their mental illness – conditions which, thankfully, are no longer burdened by stigma. It no doubt also has something to do with the widespread consumer acceptance of antidepressants as a solution for their depression.

According to some estimates, depression, that most common of mental illnesses, affects one quarter of all Americans.

A March 24, 2014 report in *The Atlantic* claims Americans are awash in pills. "The use of antidepressants has increased 400 percent between 1988 and 2008. They're now one of the three most-prescribed categories of drugs, coming in right after painkillers and cholesterol medications".

The situation, it seems, is little better elsewhere in the Western world. In the UK, for example, more than 50 million prescriptions for antidepressants are written every year if latest estimates are correct.

This figure is "staggeringly high," according to an article in *The Guardian* dated April 13, 2014. It quotes Dr Matthijs Muijen, head of mental health at the World Health Organization Europe, as saying prescription levels have gone through the roof, claiming "There's a degree of fashion about antidepressants".

Dr Muijen admits his worry is "We are medicalising all forms of sadness in the belief that antidepressants are a safe drug that you just prescribe".

In a report dated August 3, 2013, *BBC News* asks the question: "Is England a nation on anti-depressants?" It also asks why we are seeing "such huge and rising numbers of people" regularly taking anti-depressants when GPs are advised to prescribe them only for more seriously ill patients.

The report continues, "In some places the number of patients prescribed anti-depressants exceeds the number of people in that area estimated to suffer from depression and anxiety by the NHS England's Psychiatric Morbidity Survey (PMS)".

On June 21, 2013, *Healthline News* reported that a Mayo Clinic study found that nearly 70% of Americans are prescribed at least one medication, with antidepressants (along with antibiotics and opioids) topping the list.

The article quotes the National Alliance on Mental Illness as estimating one in four Americans experience a mental health disorder, such as depression or anxiety, in a given year. "Typical first-line treatments for mental health issues are medication and some type of psychotherapy…Critics who say antidepressant medications are overused often claim there is a chicken-and-egg phenomenon, saying that antidepressants are prescribed for normal human reactions to life events, leading to a lasting diagnosis of mental illness".

The article concludes, "However, as the public mindset continues to change, there's now less stigma attached to getting help for mental disorders, which may help explain the rise in antidepressant use".

Predictably, the *Psychiatric Times*, whose audience is American psychiatrists and mental health professionals, doesn't agree that antidepressants are overprescribed in the US. In an article dated September 1, 2014, that publication's editor-in-chief Ronald W. Pies, MD, reports that, "by and large", he doesn't agree with the allegation that America has become a kind of *Prozac Nation* – a none-too-subtle reference to the title of Elizabeth Wurtzel's 1994 memoirs perhaps.

"In many respects, the claim that 'too many Americans are taking antidepressants' is a myth," according to Dr. Pies. "…To be sure: in some primary care settings, antidepressants are prescribed too casually; after too little evaluation time; and for instances of normal stress or everyday sadness, rather than for MDD (major depressive disorder)," he says.

"And, in my experience, antidepressants are vastly over-prescribed for patients with bipolar disorder, where these drugs often do more harm than good: mood stabilizers, such as lithium, are safer and more effective in bipolar disorder. But these kernels of truth are concealed within a very large pile of chaff".

Dr. Pies continues, "For example, the media often report that antidepressant use in the United States has 'gone up by 400%' in recent years—and that's probably true…But the actual percentage of Americans 12 years or older taking antidepressants is about 11%—a large proportion of the population, for sure, but not exactly Prozac Nation".

So, though Dr. Pies – and by default *Psychiatric Times* and no doubt the majority of psychiatric professionals in the US – disputes the allegation that America has become a kind of *Prozac Nation*, there seems to be a reluctant acknowledgement that antidepressants are vastly over-prescribed for patients suffering one type of mental illness at least, and that it's probably true that antidepressant use has risen 400% in the US.

If that doesn't constitute a *Prozac Nation*, not sure what does…

Washington D.C. writer Brendan L. Smith, reporting on the American Psychological Association's website in June 2012, reports that research shows that all too often, Americans are taking medications that may not work or that may be inappropriate for their mental health problems.

Smith observes that writing a prescription to treat a mental health disorder is easy, but it may not always be the safest or most effective route for patients, according to some recent studies and a growing chorus of voices concerned about the rapid rise in the prescription of psychotropic drugs.

"Today, patients often receive psychotropic medications without being evaluated by a mental health professional, according to…the Centers for Disease Control and Prevention. Many Americans visit their primary-care physicians and may walk away with a prescription for an antidepressant or other drugs without being aware of other evidence-based treatments…that might work better for them without the risk of side effects".

Smith quotes Steven Hollon, PhD, a psychology professor at Vanderbilt University, as saying at least half the folks who are being treated with antidepressants aren't benefiting from the active pharmacological effects of the drugs themselves but from a placebo effect. "If people knew more," Hollon says, "I think they would be a little less likely to go down the medication path than the psychosocial treatment path".

Smith claims *Prozac* opened the floodgates. "Since the launch of Prozac, antidepressant use has quadrupled in the United States…Antidepressants are the second most commonly prescribed drug in the United States, just after cholesterol-lowering drugs".

Smith also quotes Daniel Carlat, MD, associate clinical professor of psychiatry at Tufts University, as saying health insurance reimbursements are higher and easier to obtain for drug treatment than therapy, which has contributed to the increase in psychotropic drug sales.

"There is a huge financial incentive for psychiatrists to prescribe instead of doing psychotherapy," Dr. Carlat says. "You can make two, three, four times as much money being a prescriber than a therapist".

> *"As James Surowiecki noted in a New Yorker article,
> given a choice between developing antibiotics that
> people will take every day for two weeks and
> antidepressants that people will take every day forever,
> drug companies not surprisingly opt for the latter.
> Although a few antibiotics have been toughened up a bit,
> the pharmaceutical industry hasn't given us an entirely
> new antibiotic since the 1970s."*
>
> – Bill Bryson, A Short History of Nearly Everything

The prescribing of antidepressants to children is a real hot potato – and rightly so.

On *MedicineNet.com*, medical author Barbara K. Hecht, PhD, and medical editor Frederick Hecht, M.D., advise subscribers that the British Government has warned that the antidepression drug *Effexor* should not be taken by children.

Furthermore, they report, "Now the UK is advising against the prescription of all antidepressant drugs (selective serotonin reuptake inhibitors or SSRIs) for children, with the exception of *Prozac*, because these drugs increase the risk of suicide".

Their report includes a statement by the Medicines and Healthcare Products Regulatory Agency (MHRA). It reads as follows:

"Use of Selective Serotonin Reuptake Inhibitors (SSRIs) in children and adolescents with major depressive disorder (MDD) - only fluoxetine (Prozac) shown to have a favourable balance of risks and benefits for the treatment of MDD in the under 18s.

"On the basis of a review of the safety and efficacy of the SSRI class in the treatment of paediatric major depressive disorder undertaken by the Expert Working Group of the Committee on Safety of Medicines (CSM), the CSM has advised that the balance of risks and benefits for the treatment of major depressive disorder in under 18s is judged to be unfavourable for sertraline (Zoloft), citalopram (Celexa) and escitalopram (Lexapro) and unassessable for fluvoxamine (Luvox)".

Overmedication of children diagnosed – and often *misdiagnosed* or even *not* diagnosed – with ADHD (Attention Deficit Hyperactivity

Disorder) has also, it seems, reached alarming levels, and the public debate has been as vocal as that surrounding the issue of overprescribing antidepressants.

By some estimates, around four million children in the US have been diagnosed with ADHD and more than half of them have been prescribed drugs. This despite the fact there are very real concerns about the impact the drugs have on growth and brain development – especially in preschoolers.

One who has had something to say on this matter of late is Dr. Nancy Rappaport, a certified child and adolescent psychiatrist at Cambridge Health Alliance and an associate professor of psychiatry at Harvard Medical School. In a *Washington Post* article dated June 4, 2014, and headed 'We are overmedicating America's poorest kids,' she claims that thousands of children between the ages of two and three are being prescribed stimulants like *Ritalin* or *Adderall* for ADHD even though the medicine's safety and effectiveness has barely been explored in that age group.

Dr. Rappaport says she finds it even more troubling that a disproportionate number of those children were on Medicaid, which to her is an indicator of poverty. "That," she says, "is the huge red flag".

Referring to her experience as a child psychiatrist, working with at-risk children for more than 20 years, she points out the simple fact is that underprivileged children often grow up in home environments that lead to troubling behavior.

"To the untrained observer, it looks as if these children suffer from ADHD. But they don't need medicine. They need stability and support".

This raises the obvious question: Why are physicians prescribing potentially harmful drugs instead of recommending family-based support services for toddlers who display ADHD symptoms and disruptive behavior?

Dr. Rappaport asks this very question. She says, "Medication may be judiciously used to help ADHD when a biological illness is truly present, but true ADHD cannot be differentiated from other problems at such young ages. We owe it to our children to give the consistent message that we will do whatever it takes to foster their development. And that doesn't always mean prescribing a pill".

Amen to that.

It's a fact that in this modern era most of us look for a quick fix for whatever ails us or for whatever ails our children. Our willingness to pop a pill in order to get a good night's sleep or to ease a queasy tummy or to clear a foggy head or to…(the list goes on) is frightening. Even more so when we pass such *quick fix* ideas onto our children.

We seem very willing to overlook the fact that all drugs – prescribed or otherwise – have side-effects. Sometimes deadly side-effects, often unhealthy or otherwise undesirable side-effects.

We also overlook the fact that oftentimes there's a simple, readily available, natural remedy available for those day-to-day ailments we encounter.

For example, physical exercise has long been recognized as an effective way to combat depression. Not for all, granted, but, we suspect, for many.

The Atlantic article referred to earlier reports that a growing body of research suggests that exercise is one of its best cures for depression. It claims a randomized controlled trial showed that depressed adults who took part in aerobic exercise improved as much as those treated with *Zoloft*, and a recommendation was made that physicians counsel their depressed patients to try it.

A later study looked at 127 depressed people who hadn't experienced relief from a commonly used antidepressant and found that exercise led 30% of them into remission – a result described "as good as, or better than" drugs alone.

The article continues, "Though we don't know exactly how any antidepressant works, we think exercise combats depression by enhancing endorphins: natural chemicals that act like morphine and other painkillers. There's also a theory that aerobic activity boosts norepinephrine, a neurotransmitter that plays a role in mood. And like antidepressants, exercise helps the brain grow new neurons".

The article concludes that "this powerful, non-drug treatment" hasn't yet become a mainstream remedy. Why not? And why are so many people still popping pills?

We suspect the conclusion speaks volumes about the state of our mental health services and infrastructure, the physician reimbursement system (more about doctors' kickbacks coming up) and the alacrity with which doctors dispense prescription drugs ahead of advising on diet, exercise and other lifestyle changes.

Regrettably, it also speaks volumes about our unwillingness to take responsibility for, and control of, our own health, preferring, instead, to entrust that to our family doctor.

Chapter 8

Kickbacks for doctors

"The vast majority of curricula that are taught in medical schools in this country (USA) were put together by organizations that were founded by, or are funded by, pharmaceutical companies."

–T.C. Hale, natural health expert

It was Cicero who said, "In nothing do men more nearly approach the gods than in giving health to men." Certainly, the medical profession, in its purest form, is a noble one. And doctors are clearly at the apex of the profession.

We have no wish to denigrate doctors, or to denigrate anyone who devotes their life to helping fellow man. However, it would be remiss of us not to bring your attention to some, shall we say, gaps in the system – gaps that allow doctors to abuse their position if they are so inclined.

And we stress that those who do (abuse their position) are very much in the minority. That said, the number of doctors who have brought their profession into disrepute, worldwide, is staggeringly high. Certainly far too many for so noble a profession, we would argue.

The following report was aired by *BBC News* on November 6, 2014: "Until recently, paying bribes to doctors to prescribe their drugs was commonplace at big pharmas, although the practice is now generally frowned upon and illegal in many places. GSK (GlaxoSmithKline) was fined $490m in China in September for bribery and has been accused of similar practices in Poland and the Middle East.

"The rules on gifts, educational grants and sponsoring lectures, for example, are less clear cut, and these practices remain commonplace in the US. Indeed a recent study found that doctors in the US receiving payments from pharma companies were twice as likely to prescribe their drugs.

"This may well exacerbate the problem of overspending on drugs by governments. A recent study by Prescribing Analytics suggested that the UK's National Health Service could save up to £1bn a year by doctors switching from branded to equally effective generic versions of the drugs".

> *"Isn't it a bit unnerving that doctors call what they do practice?"*
>
> *–Grammy-winning American actor/author George Carlin*

The "recent study" referred to by *BBC News* was a detailed 61-page report compiled by the University of California, San Diego (UCSD), and dated January 2014.

This report starts out with the comment that "While rent-seeking behavior may not be surprising generally, that financial conflicts of interest could influence physicians' advice might be less expected. For one, doctors are highly paid, with most falling in the top 5% of the income distribution within the US".

The UCSD report continues, "When drug companies have financial relationships with physicians, medical decisions may be influenced by pecuniary motives not directly related to patient health…

"We find that men are over twice as sensitive to payments as women. This confirms experimental and field evidence suggesting that women are, on average, more honest and less corruptible than men".

The report's conclusion is that "Using data from twelve drug companies, more than 330,000 physicians and nearly one billion prescriptions, we find that when a drug company pays a doctor he is more likely to prescribe that company's drug.

"Whether these results are surprising likely depends on whether one views a physician – and her opinions – as sacrosanct. To a cynical reader, perhaps the presence of influence is self-evident from payments: after all, if payments from firms to doctors did not change doctor behavior, why would profit-maximizing firms choose to make them in the first place?

"While this view seems sensible from an economist's perspective, it ignores the fact that payments may reflect (rather than cause) the opinions of physicians or represent valuable transfers of information from firms to doctors. Given that the balance of our evidence is best explained by either persuasive advertising from drug companies or rent-seeking behavior from doctors, to a less-cynical reader our findings suggest a consideration of outside influences when taking in medical advice".

Reading the UCSD report, we got the feeling the researchers were choosing their words very carefully – as they should of course. However, the distinct impression we were left with was they went above and beyond to ensure that criticism of the medical profession was presented in the most benign and inoffensive terms possible. But we concede that could be a cynical view.

> *"The purpose of a doctor or any human in general should not be to simply delay the death of the patient, but to increase the person's quality of life."*
>
> *–Patch Adams*

A US Federal Government report unveiled in September 2014, detailing 4.4 million payments made to doctors and teaching hospitals by pharmaceutical and medical device companies sheds more light on the vexing *kickbacks* issue.

ProPublica.com, a watchdog site that prides itself on providing "journalism in the public interest," analyzes the Federal Government report in an article dated September 30, 2014 by award-winning reporter Charles Ornstein.

Incidentally, the site's management advises subscribers that "ProPublica is investigating the financial ties between the medical community and the drug and device industry," and "in 2010, ProPublica compiled the list of payments that drug companies make to physicians and built a publicly searchable database so that patients could look up their doctors".

We quote Charles Ornstein quite freely in this chapter, so it's worth sharing his credentials with you. According to Wikipedia, Ornstein is a graduate of the University of Pennsylvania and was a reporter for the Washington bureau of *The Dallas Morning News* and the *Los Angeles Times*; he was a Media Fellow with the Henry J. Kaiser Family Foundation and is vice president of the Association of Health Care Journalists; he shared the 2005 Pulitzer Prize for Public Service, citing "courageous, exhaustively researched series exposing deadly medical problems and racial injustice at a major public hospital".

In his *ProPublica* column, Ornstein points out that the Federal Government's "new trove of data" covers the period August to December 2013. He writes, "According to officials from the Centers for Medicare and Medicaid Services, companies spent a total of $3.5 billion during that period on 546,000 individual physicians and almost 1,360 teaching hospitals".

Under the heading 'Where Did the Payments Go?', Ornstein provides the following breakdown of general payments (that drug companies make to physicians) by category. (Amounts in US dollars):

Royalty or licence payments – $302m; promotional speaking – $202.6m; consulting fees – $158.2m; food and beverage – $92.8m; travel and lodging – $74.1m; grants – $38.1m; education – $26.7m; honoraria – $25.5m; gifts – $19.2m; the balance of payments included space rental, charitable contributions and entertainment. (Payments *excluded* research or fees to physician owners of a company).

Ornstein states, "Similarly, companies reported payments associated with particular drugs in different ways. The expensive drug Acthar, which is marketed for a variety of different conditions, is listed under at least eight different name variations…There is one drug simply listed as 'KNEES' and another as 'Foot and Ankle'."

One of his most alarming observations is that more than 1.7 million records did *not* include the names of the doctors or hospitals that received the payments. By his calculation, that amounts to 40% of the payments.

Ornstein also calculates the redactions were even more extensive. "About 64 percent of the total spending by companies wasn't attributable to a particular doctor or hospital (the names, addresses and other identifying information were removed)".

He concludes, "Doctors were paid for more than 200,000 trips by companies in the last five months of the year…Their top destinations were Toronto, Copenhagen, Amsterdam, Paris and Barcelona. Drug and device makers paid for doctors to travel to about 80 countries in all".

"An apple a day, if well aimed, keeps the doctor away."

–P.G. Wodehouse

Ornstein also figures in an item *CBS News* ran on March 4, 2014. Headed 'Does your doctor have ties to Big Pharma,' the report states, "Big pharma routinely pays doctors to promote its products, but soon patients will be able to get a clearer picture about a doctor's possible connections to the companies that make the drugs they may prescribe".

The report continues, "The practice of pharmaceutical companies working with doctors to develop new medications to treat conditions and help promote those medications has been in place for decades, but Ornstein, who is investigating this practice, says, 'The promotion part has gotten a lot of attention in recent years because drug companies have paid hundreds of millions and sometimes billions of dollars to settle lawsuits that have accused them of improper marketing and giving kickbacks to doctors'."

The same report addresses the all-important issue of trust – trust between patient and doctor. As Ornstein points out, "When you go to your doctor, you trust that the doctor is giving the best medication for you, but there's a lot of different interests that your doctor has to take in mind in prescribing you drugs".

In response, Matthew Bennett, senior vice president of the Pharmaceutical Research and Manufacturers of America, is reported by *CBS News* as saying the discovery of new and improved medicines is dependent on research collaborations between physicians and biopharmaceutical companies. "Clinical trials sponsored by biopharmaceutical companies have led to breakthroughs for people suffering from cancer and other life-threatening diseases".

We don't doubt there's some truth to that, but it doesn't address the concerns held by many – that it's illegal to give kickbacks to doctors to prescribe drugs.

Of equal concern to us is that it is *legal* for pharmaceutical companies to give money to doctors to help promote their drugs. How tempting it must be for doctors to put impartiality aside when recommending certain drugs to patients. And how tempting it must be for unscrupulous doctors to recommend lesser or inferior drugs, knowing promotional payments – aka *kickbacks* – are on offer.

As Ornstein advised *CBS News*, "Some doctors make tens of thousands or hundreds of thousands of dollars a year beyond their normal practice just for working with the industry".

Yes, you read that right: *tens of thousands or hundreds of thousands of dollars a year beyond their normal practice.*

Of course, this is nothing new. The practice has been around for ages, but we've limited the bulk of our research to cases dating back to the mid-2000's.

One earlier case that caught our attention was reported by *New York Times* on March 3, 2009. Under the heading 'Crackdown on Doctors Who Take Kickbacks,' reporter Gardiner Harris writes, "Federal health officials and prosecutors, frustrated that they have been unable to stop illegal kickbacks to doctors from drug and device companies, are investigating doctors who take money for using these products".

Harris states, "For years, prosecutors rarely pursued doctors because they believed that juries would sympathize with respected clinicians. But within a few months, officials plan to file civil and criminal charges against a number of surgeons who they say demanded profitable consulting agreements from device makers in exchange for using their products.

"The move against doctors is part of a diverse campaign to curb industry marketing tactics that enrich doctors but increase health care costs and sometimes endanger patients. Taken together, the new measures are likely to transform the relationship between medicine and industry".

Harris concludes with a quote by the US attorney, Mr Sullivan, who said, "Officials hoped to send a strong message to doctors," and "I have been shocked at what appears to be willful blindness by folks in the physician community to the criminal conduct that corrupts the patient-physician relationship".

"Doctors put drugs of which they know little into bodies of which they know less for diseases of which they know nothing at all."

–Voltaire

A *Washington Post* report that was picked up by media around the world in February 2015 points out that Americans spent $329 billion, or approximately $1000 per person, on prescription drugs in 2013. Quoting John Oliver, of the *Last Week Tonight* show as its source, the newspaper reports that nine out of the 10 big pharmaceutical companies spend less on research than on marketing. (A lot less as it turns out).

The report confirms that US television channels screen ads for pharmaceutical products that require a doctor's prescriptions. It concludes with the following quote from Oliver: "Ask your doctor today if he's taking pharmaceutical money (then ask) what the money is for…Then ask yourself if you're satisfied with that answer".

Little mention has been made thus far of kickbacks physicians receive from medical equipment manufacturers and suppliers. As with the relationship between the pharmaceutical companies and doctors, business dealings between medical equipment representatives and doctors are worthy of scrutiny.

There's no doubt that an honest relationship between these two parties makes for a win-win for all. There's potential to progress science and technology, and to help ensure the health and safety of patients. However, the key word here is *honest*. For there is potential for fraud and abuse, and, as it turns out, some are taking advantage of this.

In America, this sad state of affairs prompted the US Government to introduce the federal *Anti-kickback Statute*, which imposes criminal penalties on anyone soliciting, receiving, offering or paying any remuneration for any item or service, directly or indirectly, to anyone involved in a federal healthcare program.

Judging by the number of confirmed abuses of that statute, it appears it hasn't worked.

US law firm Phillips and Cohen, which advertises itself as

"Representing whistleblowers across the nation and around the world," observes that the sales and marketing tactics used by medical device companies, "such as lucrative consulting agreements with doctors and off-label marketing" could violate the False Claims Act and "both the pharmaceutical and medical device industries follow some of the same sales and marketing practices".

On its website, Phillips and Cohen states that sales representatives and their companies in "highly lucrative, competitive segments of the medical device industry" probably face the greatest pressure to win market share.

"There may be more pressure to offer kickbacks to doctors to win their business. This includes markets for **implantable cardioverter defibrillators and pacemakers,** stents, prosthetic heart valves and other cardiac implant devices; orthopedic implants (including artificial hips and artificial knees); spinal disks; cochlear implants; and robotic surgery machines".

Stating the obvious, the posting concludes that payments to physicians could be considered improper financial inducements if they could influence the doctors' choices. "Free vacations, unrestricted grants and consulting agreements could be considered kickbacks as they might influence doctors' choices of implants and other medical devices".

For a snapshot of just how widespread corruption is within the medical equipment supply sector, and unfortunately, amongst their clients within the medical profession, take a look at the website of New York trial lawyer John Howley, Esq. It lists numerous examples of historic kickbacks deemed illegal under the Anti-kickback Statute and subsequently successfully prosecuted.

These examples include the case of a physician and the owner of a medical supply company pleading guilty to a conspiracy to defraud Medicare by submitting false claims for power wheelchairs, a durable medical equipment (DME) supplier being imprisoned for paying kickbacks to co-conspirators for medical prescriptions and a doctor pleading guilty to accepting kickbacks from the makers of power wheelchairs and other DME.

Pride of place on Howley's site goes to the $42 million settlement involving American medical device manufacturer Orthofix, Inc., which was (*reportedly*) formally convicted and sentenced for criminal violations related to its obstruction of a federal audit of the company's bone growth stimulator medical devices.

It's not clear what involvement Howley's firm had, if any, with this particular settlement. However, the media page of the US Attorney's Office website reports that "Orthofix manipulated patients' medical records and tried to hide its misconduct from federal investigators, in order to defraud the Medicare program". It quotes US Attorney Carmen M. Ortiz as saying, "The Orthofix investigation, which has resulted in the conviction of six individuals so far, including a high-ranking executive, reinforces this office's historic commitment to protecting taxpayers from health care fraud".

Hopefully, this insight into doctors' kickbacks from the likes of Big Pharma and the medical equipment suppliers hasn't destroyed your faith in your family doctor. We stress that those who succumb to the temptations on offer are in the minority and so, statistically speaking, we'd like to think there's a very small chance your doctor is one of the culprits.

However, if you are tempted to consider alternatives (to conventional medicine) then upcoming chapters on alternative health and natural medicine may well be of interest...

CHAPTER 9

Conspiring to quash alternative medicines

*"The doctor of the future will give no medication, but
will interest his patients in the care of the human frame,
diet and in the cause and prevention of disease."*

–*Thomas Edison*

If the Medical Industrial Complex is the Devil in healthcare, then natural or alternative medicine would probably be God.

Natural medicine... Sounds like an oxymoron doesn't it? Given the dictionary interpretation of *medicine* is *drug* or *medication*, little wonder *natural medicine* sounds contradictory. However, it's no secret that *natural medicine* – like *alternative health* – is (once more) a widely used, well understood term and is a practice that has legions of followers the world over. And those legions are increasing – much to the consternation of mainstream medicine.

Many in the medical fraternity instantly label treatments in the traditional, natural or holistic health fields as *quackery*. This word is even used to describe Traditional Chinese Medicine (TCM) and the Indian Ayurveda – two medical systems which are far older than Western medicine and globally just as popular.

One sign that the Medical Industrial Complex may view natural or alternative medicine as a financial threat is the sweeping law changes it has forced upon the alternative health market in recent years.

Today, most nations now have laws requiring any health substance with medicinal claims to be legally defined as "drugs." This includes herbal remedies and various other *non-drug* medicines of natural origins. Critics say such laws prevent wider distribution of natural health products and give Big Pharma ever more control.

In the US, these laws are monitored by the FDA (the Food and Drug Administration), an organization which critics argue is at the very top of the Medical Industrial Complex. That's right folks, the same FDA that allows genetically-modified Monsanto organisms in your food supply and the same FDA that allows your kids to consume Aspartame in soft drinks is the organization responsible for telling Americans how they can and cannot treat their illnesses.

It has been repeatedly argued by natural health proponents that major pharmaceutical companies, along with their supportive cronies in government, conspired to pass these laws to force the public to only use modern medicines that are pharmacological, patented or patentable, and profitable.

Call us crazy, but we think any product with 100% natural and non-synthetic ingredients such as those derived from the likes of herbs, flowers, fruits and roots should be in a totally separate category to synthetic, laboratory-made pharmaceutical drugs.

> *"We each have the innate ability to heal ourselves. To empower ourselves with natural solutions, instead of succumbing to life-altering chemicals. There's a time and place for pharmaceuticals, but it shouldn't be the first answer, nor the only form of treatment."*
>
> *–American wellness coach and author Dana Arcuri*

Many alternative health researchers also claim that little funding is granted for research into natural or traditional cures because Big Pharma cannot patent plants or anything else that occurs organically in nature.

One such example is the work of high-profile American chemist and Nobel Prize recipient Linus Pauling (1901-1994). He received no support from the medical establishment for radical health discoveries (he claimed) he discovered when experimenting with mega-doses of Vitamin C. Despite his illustrious credentials, Pauling was also labeled a quack for his claims that the natural, *unpatentable* Vitamin C could cure a whole host of diseases, including cancer.

However, it appears Pauling may have the last laugh, albeit posthumously. Several high profile studies in the last few years suggest his theories on high dose Vitamin C being an effective anticancer agent may indeed be correct.

America's National Cancer Institute (NCI) provides a brief history of the **use of high-dose Vitamin C as a complementary and alternative treatment for cancer on its website, pointing out that** "High-dose vitamin C has been studied as a treatment for patients with cancer since the 1970s".

NCI states, "A Scottish surgeon named Ewan Cameron worked with…Linus Pauling to study the possible benefits of vitamin C therapy in clinical trials of cancer patients in the late 1970s and early 1980's" and "In the 1970's, it was proposed that high-dose ascorbic acid could help build resistance to disease or infection and possibly treat cancer".

Interestingly, the institute concedes, "Laboratory studies have shown…treatment with high-dose vitamin C slowed the growth and spread of prostate, pancreatic, liver, colon, malignant mesothelioma, neuroblastoma, and other types of cancer cells," and "combining high-dose vitamin C with certain types of chemotherapy may be more effective than chemotherapy alone".

NCI refers to another laboratory study that "suggested that combining high-dose vitamin C with radiation therapy killed more glioblastoma multiforme cells than radiation therapy alone".

The institute advises that "The FDA has not approved the use of high-dose vitamin C as a treatment for cancer or any other medical condition" and "Because dietary supplements are regulated as foods, not as drugs, FDA approval is not required unless specific claims about disease prevention or treatment are made".

However, it seems the door remains open at least. As NCI concedes, "More studies of combining high-dose IV vitamin C with other drugs are in progress".

On October 12, 2014, Television New Zealand's *'Sunday'* current affairs program advised viewers that ground breaking research at Otago University had revealed Vitamin C may be a useful tool in cancer treatment.

The report states, "Professor Margreet Vissers has told the Sunday Programme Vitamin C is unlikely to provide a miracle cure. However it could be used alongside other therapies. 'We think Vitamin C is potentially another tool in the toolbox of anti-cancer treatments.'

"Lab tests at Otago showed tumours with higher levels of Vitamin C were less aggressive and slower to grow than ones with lower levels of the vitamin. A number of doctors around the country have been running centres which offer the treatment to patients as an alternative or a complement to chemotherapy and radio therapy. They are using high level doses of Vitamin C by intravenous infusion to attack the tumours".

Vissers also says, "What we want to find out…is if we increase the amount of Vitamin C is that going to slow the tumour growth as well? We suspect it will".

On May 6, 2014, under the heading 'Taking on Big C with Vitamin C,' the New Zealand newspaper *The Northern Advocate* reported on the incredible case of policeman Anton Kuraia, a family man and cancer patient "who was given only weeks to live" after unsuccessful chemotherapy.

The article reads, "The medical experts described it as 'wall to wall' cancer and after two months of intensive chemotherapy there was little improvement. Anton Kuraia was sent home from hospital with weeks to live and told he would slip into a coma and die.

"The 43-year-old Whangarei policeman and father of three was left shattered and broken. 'I remember asking my oncology doctor if there was anything I could do, anything at all. But it was made clear that there were no other options and that certain death would be upon me'."

The article continues, "Anton got on the internet and googled vitamin C".

Anton is quoted as saying, "I naturally looked into high dose vitamin C, therapies and supplements on the other side of the pharmaceutical fence. Why is it that we call everything that isn't conventional medicine 'alternative'? When you reflect on the simple methodology of alternatives you soon discover that the term 'naturals' is a clearer description. Naturals support, detoxify and gently encourage the body to create an environment in which cancer struggles to survive."

Apparently, Anton's diet was given a major overhaul, with sugar being a definite no-go food.

"Fresh vegetable and fruit smoothies became the order of the day as he followed a blood type diet. The high dose liquid form of vitamin C is 90g of clear liquid taken intravenously to bypass the gut…The sessions cost $200 each.

"After 10 weeks of healthy eating and infusions - two weeks longer than experts had predicted he would live - Anton was feeling better and agreed to have a bone marrow biopsy. The results revealed the cancer had dwindled to less than one per cent. The cancer was in complete remission".

It's abundantly clear not everyone agrees that Vitamin C may be an effective anticancer agent. On its website, the American Cancer Society states, "Clinical trials of high doses vitamin C as a treatment for cancer have not shown any benefit." And it warns, "High doses of vitamin C can cause side effects in some people".

To be fair, high doses of *anything* can cause side effects – even death – if consumers overdo it. (Try eating a truckload of apples and see how you feel).

However, the American Cancer Society's point is taken: high doses of Vitamin C can cause side effects and, it seems, the jury's still out on the effectiveness, or otherwise, of this vitamin as an anticancer agent.

The society does acknowledge that "Some claim that the vitamin can prevent a variety of cancers from developing, including lung, prostate, bladder, breast, cervical, intestinal, esophageal, stomach, pancreatic, and salivary gland cancers, as well as leukemia and non-Hodgkin's lymphoma. Vitamin C is also said to prevent tumors from spreading, help the body heal after cancer surgery, enhance the effects of certain anti-cancer drugs, and reduce the toxic effects of other drugs used in chemotherapy".

And while the society acknowledges that "people with higher blood levels of vitamin C tend to have a lesser risk of developing cancer than do people with lower levels," it categorically states, "Studies that observed large groups or people and clinical trials of vitamin C supplements have not shown the same strong protective effects against cancer".

The American Cancer Society also quotes a 2000 National Academy of Sciences report as saying, "There is not enough evidence to support claims that taking high doses of antioxidants (such as vitamins C and E, selenium, and beta carotene) can prevent chronic diseases".

Certainly, some doctors recommend high doses of vitamin C

supplements to protect patients against, and to treat, the common cold. However, it does seem that few doctors are prepared to accept that high doses of Vitamin C may be an effective anticancer agent.

> *"Each patient carries his own doctor inside him."*
>
> –Norman Cousins, Author of Anatomy of an Illness

The basis of many a drug or medicine, of course, is a plant or plants. These plants range from herbs, flowers, roots and leaves to common and uncommon weeds.

According to one (unconfirmed) source, there are 120 or more important drugs currently in use that have been sourced from plants. These drugs include the likes of *morphine, camphor, papain, hesperidin, quinine, codein, ephedrine, strychnine* and *thymol.*

Under the heading 'Plant based drugs and medicines,' the natural health site *Rain-tree.com* features an interesting article by alternative health commentator Leslie Taylor on this very subject.

Taylor says the plant chemical quinine "which was discovered in a rainforest tree (*Cinchona ledgeriana*) over 100 years ago" is a good example of a plant that has been chemically copied or synthesized by laboratories and is a good example of a drug in which no plant materials have been used in its manufacture.

The article continues, "For many years the quinine chemical was extracted from the bark of this tree and processed into pills to treat malaria. Then a scientist was able to synthesize or copy this plant alkaloid into a chemical drug without using the original tree bark for manufacturing the drug. Today, all quinine drugs sold are manufactured chemically without the use of any tree bark".

This got us thinking... How many plants are being unnecessarily synthesized and sold over the counter as wonder drugs to an unsuspecting public?

Remember, the pharmaceutical companies cannot patent anything that occurs organically in nature. So there's no incentive for them to harvest, develop and sell herbs, leaves or any other plants. Far more profitable to synthesize or copy those plants, patent the resulting drugs and medicines, and then sell them.

What if those patented drugs and medicines are less effective in the treatment of diseases and illnesses than the actual plants they are derived from? Think of the cost-savings – not to mention the health benefits to be gained by ingesting or applying natural substances as opposed to toxic chemicals.

Has that occurred to anyone else?

It occurred to us during our research for this book when someone very close to us – let's call him *Mr X* – sought treatment for the very common solar keratosis, or sunspots, at a local skin clinic. Mr X was attracted by the clinic's advertised use of a new drug, *Picato*, which is an extract of milkweed – also known as radium weed and cancer weed.

Said to work considerably faster than other topical medications, dosing is completed in just two to three days (compared to two to four weeks for competitive products). As you can imagine, the skin's reaction to such a powerful medication is quite dramatic. Users suffer drastic reddening of the skin and often painful blisters.

Turns out the *Picato* treatment is very expensive – and quite toxic. Like the better known and more widely used *Efudex* treatment (for sunspots), *Picato* is potentially harmful to the liver and therefore the recommended dosage per treatment is wisely limited.

The logic put forward by the skin specialists concerned is the alternative (to *Picato* or *Efudex*) could be fatal. They refer of course to deadly melanoma or skin cancer.

That logic's hard to argue with. But Mr X wondered why he couldn't simply use milkweed to treat his sunspots. So he did some research.

Turns out milkweed in its natural form is very effective for treating sunspots and potential skin cancers. Users simply break the stem of the plant and apply the milky sap to the skin.

Of course, plants can be toxic, too, and milkweed's no exception – depending on the variety. For starters, like *Picato* and *Efudex*, it must not come into contact with the eyes.

The US Department of Agriculture (USDA) warns that "Milkweed may be toxic when taken internally." On its website, USDA reports that Native Americans used milkweed as a food source, and several tribes used the sap to remove warts, for ringworm, and for bee stings.

However, it was a *Daily Mail* article that clinched it for Mr X. Dated

January 26, 2011, the article quotes scientists who claimed that the sap from milkweed "can 'kill' certain types of cancer cells" and that "it works on non-melanoma skin cancers".

The article states, "For the first time a team of scientists in Australia has carried out a clinical study of sap from *Euphorbia peplus* (milkweed), which is related to *Euphorbia* plants grown in gardens in the UK…The study of 36 patients with a total of 48 non-melanoma lesions" found that "After only one month 41 of 48 cancers had completely gone".

Mr X now treats his sunspots with milkweed, which he grows in his garden. Last we heard he's still alive and well!

That said, the Mr X case study was hardly scientific and therefore should not be used as a blueprint for managing the treatment of sunspots should you have any. As always, our advice must be: *Consult your doctor first.*

However, it does illustrate the point we were trying to make – that we suspect there are plants, vitamins (à la Vitamin C) and minerals out there that are safer, more effective and a whole heap cheaper than the toxic, synthesized alternatives being developed and marketed by the pharmaceutical companies.

If we are even half right then we'd suggest that would mean natural medicine and alternative treatments are worth exploring, right?

CHAPTER 10

Suppressed cures

As covered in our 2014 non-fiction book *The Orphan Conspiracies*, there seems to be more than enough evidence to support the claim that at least some scientific breakthroughs are suppressed.

In that book, in a chapter titled *Suppressed Science*, we cite a January 2014 *New York Times* article reporting that America's National Security Agency (NSA) uses secret technology to remotely input and alter data on computers worldwide – even when targeted PC's or laptops are not connected to the Internet. We point out that this suppressed technology, which uses radio frequencies to spy on computers, only came to the public's attention due to leaked NSA documents from former agency contractor-turned whistleblower Edward Snowden.

This begs the question: Is it a regular occurrence for governments, intelligence agencies and the military to withhold scientific breakthroughs from the public?

If so, how many other suppressed inventions exist in the world's ironclad vaults of power?

Replace the word *inventions* with *cures* and you will see what we, in our roundabout way, are driving at.

There have been numerous reports of scientific inventions that never saw the light of day even though they were perfected and ready to go on the market. Rumors of these radical inventions date back to the post-Industrial Revolution period in the late 1800's and early 1900's, and have persisted right up to and including the present day.

Unfortunately, it appears this also happens within modern medicine where cures for various illnesses mysteriously vanish or are quashed by the medical establishment.

The basic concept or theory we explore in this chapter is that there are already cures for many so-called incurable illnesses. However, they are often unpatentable (aka unprofitable or unmonitizable) and therefore blocked by multinational drug companies.

In other instances, these cures are sometimes not suppressed for financial reasons but rather for intellectual ones: such cures contradict medical academia and these cures, which are often radical and seem *non-scientific*, "do not compute" with what official science says. But a term American banker turned author Edward Drobinski coined seems relevant in this regard: "Scientific fact, until next revision". Meaning what seems to contradict science today, may make sense tomorrow, for science is perpetually evolving.

This suppression theory supports the assertion that Big Pharma needs sick people to prosper. Patients, not healthy people, are their customers. If everybody was cured of a particular illness or disease, pharmaceutical companies would lose 100% of their revenue on the products they sell for that ailment.

What all this means is because modern medicine is so heavily intertwined with the financial profits culture, it's a *sickness industry* more than it is a health industry.

There are numerous examples we could cite to support this. One of the most disturbing examples came to our attention in the form of a *CTV News* report dated November 29, 2012. Headed 'Cure for cancer found in Canada – Pharmaceutical companies turn their backs,' the televised report highlights the successful treatment of rats and mice given human cancers in a Canadian laboratory.

The drug used was *DCA* – described by the researchers involved as "an unpatentable old drug" used to treat rare inherited diseases. Those same researchers were very excited, and confident, about its potential for curing cancer in humans and were keen to secure the interest of pharmaceutical companies to take the drug to the next step.

DCA's affordability – described as costing "just pennies a dose" – no doubt accounted for some of the researchers' enthusiasm. Here, at last, was a potential cancer cure that wouldn't cost patients the earth.

Now here's the rub. Because this cheap, unpatentable, old drug "doesn't fit the business plans" of the pharmaceutical companies, they ain't interested in progressing it. In other words, Big Pharma can see no profit in developing and marketing a pennies-a-dose drug – even if it has the likely potential of saving many, many lives.

At the time of proofing this book, the *CTV* report on this disgusting state of affairs is still on YouTube and is well worth viewing.

Of course, there are two sides to every story, and, in the interests of balance, we must relay one YouTube viewer's comment on this report.

He (name withheld) says: "Even if it was true that Big Pharma doesn't want a cure for cancer, you don't need Big Pharma to get a drug out there. There are plenty of non-profit and research institutions that have the money to fund this and have no incentive for a profit. This video is too one-sided to make a judgement…If you dig deeper into this you'll find that clinical trials into humans were conducted in 2009 and did not yield the same results (as) in rats. The attack on Big Pharma is normally done by people who have no knowledge of the pharma industry and all the costs associated to create one drug".

Naïve or fair comment? You decide.

Personally, we'd be guided by former pharmacist Denis Toovey's comment in the foreword to *Medical Industrial Complex*: "There is no hiding the huge influence drug companies have on the practice of medicine which has stalled finding real cures." That from a professional who spent 40 years in the pharmaceutical industry.

As the healthcare sector is so profitable, why would anyone believe major corruption could not flourish in this industry?

When considering this question, it's important you have a grasp of the amounts of money involved in healthcare.

Keep in mind total healthcare expenditures across the world in 2013 totaled $4.5 trillion while the global prescription drug market was worth an estimated $550 billion (annually) as long ago as 2006, according to *TheMedica.com*, the respected global healthcare marketplace site.

An article on *TheMedica's* homepage states: "The USA's medical industry comprises of more than 750,000 physicians and 5,200 hospitals. USA witnesses approximately 3.8 million inpatient visits and 20 million outpatients visit on a daily basis. Furthermore, (America) has the largest workforce – i.e. one in every 11 US residents employed in the health care business."

These estimates are supported by Forbes, which puts America's NHE (National Healthcare Expenditure) for 2012 at $3 trillion. (Interesting to see a *Forbes.com* report dated January 19, 2012, quotes one economist as saying, "We don't have a debt problem in this country – we have a healthcare problem.").

Given the huge monies up for grabs in the healthcare sector, is it really that difficult to believe corruption flourishes within it?

Also, why are so many so quick to doubt that certain cures, including cancer cures, have been suppressed because of pharmaceutical companies' desire to continue profiting off the drugs they produce to manage long-term sicknesses?

Anytime so much money is at stake, we cannot underestimate the lengths certain companies and groups will go to in their pursuit of profit.

The alternative health site *NaturalSociety.com* has an intriguing post about "an ignored method of treating and preventing most diseases – so potent that it threatens the medical establishment's tyrannical monopoly".

Called *Ozone Therapy*, the treatment was, according to the article, practiced in the US from the late 19th Century through the 1940's.

The article points out that "all bacterial pathogens, viruses, and parasites are anaerobic and thrive in the absence of oxygen. In fact, they are **poisoned by oxygen.** Even cancer cells perish with abundant oxygen. **The most common and effective therapy for oxygenating is ozone therapy".**

The writer states, "But since the 1940s, the FDA and AMA have come down hard on ozone therapy in the USA…The FDA recently warned against using hyperbaric oxygen therapy".

The article continues, "Ozone therapy is currently used successfully in Germany, Spain, Russia, the Caribbean, Mexico, Cuba and other nations. The results are astounding, and there are usually no adverse effects. Ozone is normally administered as a liquid by IV or injection and as a gas through a tube placed in the anus.

"Because of potential Herxheimer reactions ('healing crisis') that can discourage one from continuing, full percentage dosages are usually not administered until the fourth session. Oxygenation techniques can be used simply to improve health with intense detoxification and blood cleansing.

"Hyperbaric oxygen therapy is often effective by placing the patient in a highly pressurized chamber of pure oxygen. It has been used successfully for autism, AIDS, and Lyme Disease".

According to *Educate-Yourself.org*, "There are a number of alternative healing therapies that work so well and cost so little…that Organized Medicine, the Food & Drug Administration, and their overlords in the Pharmaceutical Industry (The Big Three) would rather the public not know about them. The reason is obvious: Alternative, non-toxic therapies represent a potential loss of billions of dollars to allopathic (drug) medicine and drug companies".

Referring to what he calls "forbidden cures," the writer states, "At long last, however, the public's consciousness seems to have finally reached a critical mass and is now beginning to seriously question the efficacy and appropriateness of using orthodox therapies and allopathic medicine in general".

The article continues, "The Big Three have collectively engaged in a medical conspiracy for the better part of 70 years to influence legislative bodies on both the state and federal level *to create regulations that promote the use of drug medicine while simultaneously creating restrictive, controlling* mechanisms…designed to limit and stifle the availability of non-drug, alternative modalities. The conspiracy to limit and eliminate competition from non-drug therapies began with the Flexner Report of 1910".

And under the heading 'Natural Healing,' the writer says, "The patient's immune system and the immune system alone is responsible for healing and recovery from ill health. The use of drugs and vaccines represents an assault on the immune system.

"In some cases, the use of a particular drug might be a wise choice to speed healing and recovery for the patient, but the use of natural, orthomolecular therapies and substances (substances normally found in Nature) that can more effectively address the cause of the disease should be considered first because natural substances work in *harmony with Nature*. They aid and stimulate the body to truly cure itself, without the terrible millstone of drug side-effects".

The article concludes with an overview of some alternative therapies that by all accounts have demonstrated themselves to be effective and readily obtainable. They include oxidative therapies, blood-electrification and nutritional therapies – most if not all of which are opposed by mainstream medical authorities.

The Northstar Report at *nstarzone.com*, which makes the claim that "Modern medicine has been made into a god by a population of people who look to the doctors and pharmaceutical companies to save them," lists natural cures it claims the medical establishment doesn't want you to know about.

These natural "cures" include: Vitamin B-17, or laetrile, which reportedly has had "amazing results" with cancer patients; ginger, which is supposedly "highly effective in preventing and curing" heart disease, cancer, arthritis, and a variety of other illnesses; and garlic, which is claimed to be "good for virtually any disease or infection".

And last, but not least, *The Northstar Report* recommends prayer, claiming "The most important aspect of healing is faith healing".

Given the state of healthcare worldwide and the dubious conduct of various sectors of the Medical Industrial Complex, prayer may be our best bet at the end of the day.

CHAPTER 11

Finding (hiding) a cure for cancer

"The cancer industry world wide is estimated at a 200 billion dollar a year industry. There are many in various associated positions within that industry who would be without a job if that cash flow dried up suddenly with the news that there are cheaper, less harmful, and more efficacious remedies available. Big Pharmacy would virtually vanish."

–Paul Fassa. Article excerpt from Natural News, September 24, 2009.

Cancer, along with cardiovascular diseases, diabetes and chronic lung diseases, is one of the biggest natural killers. Some fatality estimates suggest as many as 20,000 cancer patients are dying worldwide every day.

By some estimates, nearly two million Americans are diagnosed with cancer annually.

According to *Mercola.com*, which promotes itself as the world's No.1 natural health site, "One person out of three will be hit with a cancer diagnosis at some time in their lives." Subscribers are urged to understand that cancer is big business.

In an article dated August 3, 2013, *Mercola.com* states, "The cancer industry is spending virtually nothing of its multi-billion dollar resources on effective prevention strategies, such as dietary guidelines, exercise and obesity education. Instead, it pours its money into *treating cancer*, not preventing or curing it. Why would they shoot their cash cow? If they can keep the well-oiled Cancer Machine running, they will continue to make massive profits on chemotherapy drugs, radiotherapy, diagnostic procedures and surgeries.

"The typical cancer patient spends $50,000 fighting the disease. Chemotherapy drugs are among the most expensive of all treatments, many ranging from $3,000 to $7,000 for a one-month supply".

The article concludes, "In spite of the enormous amounts of money funneled into cancer research today, two out of three cancer patients will be dead within five years after receiving all or part of the standard cancer treatment trinity—surgery, radiotherapy and chemotherapy."

There's no doubt, in the last few decades hundreds of billions of dollars have been spent internationally on cancer research. In the US alone, since President Nixon launched his 'War on Cancer' program in 1971, tens of billions in government funding have been granted to cancer researchers.

And when a cancer cure is finally found it will save millions of lives and will be the medical discovery of the era.

However, there are theories out there which suggest there has already been a cure, or many cures, discovered for cancer. These popular theories suggest the Medical Industrial Complex have a huge financial incentive to suppress cures so they can continue to provide their own costly treatments for cancer patients.

If true, that would be a callous and unforgiveable business model, unnecessarily costing countless lives.

Of course, many if not most known (proclaimed) alternative cancer treatments are noticeably lacking in suitable testing methodology and well conducted clinical trials, and test results often haven't demonstrated significant efficacy; nor have results been published, or published in appropriate publications at least.

According to Wikipedia, "A 2006 systematic review of 214 articles covering 198 clinical trials of alternative cancer treatments concluded that almost none conducted dose-ranging studies, which are necessary to ensure that the patients are being given a useful amount of the treatment. These kinds of treatments appear and vanish frequently, and have throughout history".

The medical establishment has identified and branded as ineffective numerous alternative therapies to treat and prevent cancer. These include: homeopathy, naturopathy, herbalism, holistic medicine and aromatherapy.

Similarly, many other treatments have been put down by the establishment. To name but a few, these include light therapy and other energy-based treatments, fasting and other diet-based treatments, cannabis and other plant-based treatments, colon cleansing and other physical procedures, and faith healing and other such spiritual measures.

There's no disputing that the alternative (cancer treatment) route is littered with examples of pseudo-science, snake oil salesmen, bogus cures and failures; nor is there any disputing that in recent decades medical science has made major inroads into treating and removing cancers. You only need to look at the advances made in chemotherapy and radiation therapy, and the refinement of surgical techniques, to understand that.

However, officially at least, a cure for cancer still eludes Mankind and cancer sufferers continue to die by the millions every year.

For that reason alone, mainstream medicine should not be so quick to dismiss claims of alternative treatments and cures. After all, there are many case studies that support the theory that there has already been a cure, or many cures, discovered for cancer.

Even that respected American non-profit medical practice and research group the Mayo Clinic pays lip service at least to alternative cancer treatments. On its website, beneath the warning "Many alternative cancer treatments are unproved and some may even be dangerous," the clinic lists "10 alternative cancer treatments that are generally safe" and "have shown some promise in helping people with cancer".

Those alternative treatments (with the Mayo Clinic's abbreviated comments added) include:

- Acupuncture – "May be helpful in relieving nausea caused by chemotherapy."

- Aromatherapy – "May be helpful in relieving nausea, pain and stress."

- Exercise – "May help people with cancer live longer and improve...quality of life."

- Hypnotherapy – "May be helpful for people...who are experiencing anxiety, pain and stress."

- Massage – "Can be helpful in relieving pain."

- Meditation – "May help…by relieving anxiety and stress."

- Music therapy – "May help relieve pain and control nausea and vomiting."

- Relaxation techniques – "May be helpful in relieving anxiety and fatigue."

- Tai chi – "May help relieve stress."

- Yoga – "May provide some stress relief…improve sleep and reduce fatigue."

Hardly earth-shattering stuff. However, it's a concession at least that there is a place within mainstream medicine – no matter how small – for alternative treatments in combating cancer.

The American Cancer Society is even more conservative in its stance on alternative cancer treatments. AMC's website states that complementary or alternative cancer therapies are harder to evaluate than mainstream treatment.

AMC states, "One big concern is that, with alternative treatments, the delay in mainstream treatment can allow the cancer to grow and spread to other parts of the body. Another is that some complementary and alternative therapies have been reported to cause serious problems or even deaths. Even so, most of these problems are not reported to the FDA by the patient or family, so no one else hears about them.

"We do know that certain vitamins and minerals can increase the risk of cancer or other illnesses, especially if too much is taken. But when it happens to one person, it is very easy to miss any link between the illness and the supplement. Large groups of people must be studied to find out about a small increase in risk".

The AMC report continues, "There are those who think that treatments derived from folk remedies that have been used for thousands of years must work…just because a treatment method has been used a long time does not mean that it works…

"When scientific studies are not done, it is hard to tell what is caused by the illness and what is caused by the treatment. Herbal treatments that are given for illnesses that go away on their own may be given credit for curing the person. Or the treatment might make the person feel better for a short time but have no effect in the long run".

All good points, but it doesn't remotely change the cold, hard fact that cancer patients working within the mainstream medical system continue to succumb to the deadly disease in frightening and ever-increasing numbers. Or that no cure for cancer appears to be on the horizon within mainstream Western medicine.

What follows is a sample of alternative cancer cure theories we've unearthed as a result of conducting our own research.

In the 1920's, Canadian nurse Rene Caisse developed a natural concoction of herbs called *Essiac*. Nurse Caisse claimed it could cure cancer and she garnered many testimonials from satisfied patients said to be cancer-free after taking the product. Laboratory tests did not confirm *Essiac* offered any benefits whatsoever, but conspiracy theorists argue the lab tests were rigged and that Big Pharma flexed its muscle to shut Caisse down.

In the 1940's, German-born American physician Max Gerson (1881-1959) developed a nutrition-based cancer treatment called *Gerson Therapy*. After repeatedly claiming his therapy cured cancer, Doctor Gerson had his medical license suspended and he died while still under suspension. Although now a maligned and mostly forgotten cancer treatment in America, it remains popular in Mexico where there are Gerson clinics in operation, treating local and foreign cancer patients.

In the 1950's, American coal miner Harry Hoxsey promoted his family's century-old herbal recipe, which he touted as a cancer cure. He set up clinics in 17 states around America before all were closed down by the FDA. Hoxsey made a rare documentary film in 1957 called *You Don't Have to Die*, which detailed his cure and covered the patients he treated with it. There's a more recent documentary titled *Hoxsey: How Healing Becomes a Crime*, which chronicles his battles with what the docomakers refer to as *organized medicine*.

In the 1980's, Italian medical doctor, chemist and pharmacologist Luigi di Bella (1912-2003) claimed to have developed a cure for cancer known as *Di Bella Therapy*. The formula was a combination of vitamins, drugs and hormones.

The American Cancer Society says on its website that numerous studies showed Di Bella Therapy "may have had a negative effect compared to the outcome for similar patients receiving standard treatment". However, there are some alternative medical researchers who believe Di Bella therapy was a legitimate cancer cure that was permanently quashed by the medical establishment.

Despite the extremely negative press garnered in Italy and the rest of the world there are, or were, cancer patients who swore by Di Bella Therapy and gave testimonials. For example, on the website *BeatingCancerCenter.org* is the following statement: "For about three years, the patient has been following the Di Bella therapy without side effects, improving the quality of life and going back to work."

Luigi di Bella himself consistently stated that pharmaceutical companies were conspiring against him.

One who believes olive leaf extract can fight or even prevent cancer is a UK gentleman who is a member of our 'Underground Knowledge' discussion group on *Goodreads.com*. He speaks from some experience as he claims he battled back to full fitness after being hospitalized for four months with a rare condition. He's convinced his recovery was down to olive leaf extract, which he took in conjunction with hemp oil and Vitamin D.

Our own investigation into the merits of using olive leaf extract to combat cancer proved productive. Among the many papers published on the subject, a report by health writer Danica Collins on the *UndergroundHealthReporter.com* site claims that "The phytochemical known as oleuropein found in olive leaf extract has been shown to eliminate cancer tumors in 9 to 12 days".

Collins says, "It's no wonder that people who live in the Mediterranean area — who consume 20 times more olive oil than Americans — have half the incidences of cancer than the U.S. Both the olive leaf and olive fruit have active polyphenol properties, but in the processing of the fruit and oil, many are removed.

"Even so, olive oil contains enough polyphenols that deliver many healthful benefits. It is the olive leaf, however, that is prized for its anti-tumor, anti-microbial and anti-viral properties. And it's not just cancer that olive leaf extract has been shown to treat successfully".

She concludes, "Clinical tests conducted by the New York University School of Medicine showed that olive leaf extract is able to change the pathways of HIV-type infections as well, and may even reverse these conditions".

Collins also refers to a book titled *Olive Leaf Extract*, by Dr. Morton Walker who, she says, recommends using olive leaf extract for its miraculous effects on more than 125 infectious and chronic diseases. (We couldn't obtain a copy of this book before our own book went to press, but it sounds interesting).

The health benefits of olive leaf extract are also extoled in an article published by *Fox News* on January 23, 2013. It confirms that "Olive leaf is an especially good source of the anti-cancer compounds *apigenin* and *luteolin*, and is a source of the anti-malarial agent *cinchonine*. And *oleuropein* has also shown protective capabilities against breast cancer".

The article continues, "Olive leaf extract also acts as an anti-inflammatory. Like oxidation, inflammation is a key factor in chronic and degenerative diseases. Animal studies additionally suggest that olive leaf extract may protect against nerve damage, and may be of value in cases of stroke".

The popular science-based natural health advocacy organization Natural News, led by activist-turned-scientist Mike Adams, lists on its website "The top seven natural cures for cancer that got buried by the FDA, AMA, CDC." Detailed case studies supporting each "cure" are included in an article dated October 24, 2013 on the organization's *NaturalNews.com* site.

One of the above-mentioned case studies in particular is worth highlighting. It involves the alleged payoff of a cancer researcher to cease work on natural cures and retire in Mexico.

According to the article, the researcher, one Raymond Rife, "discovered the most promising cure for curing 'hopeless' cancer cases." He also designed and developed cutting edge microscopes and helium plasma lamps to support his research.

No surprises Rife was resented by Big Pharma and Western medicine elitists in the medical community.

The article outlines a timeline showing Rife's demise as follows:

"The AMA (American Medical Association) visits all doctors involved with Rife warning them: 'Those who don't stop using the Frequency Instruments lose their medical license.' Doctors immediately turn in their Rife Machines for fear of indictment". And (the following year) "the AMA pays (Rife's associate Dr. Arthur) Kendall over $200,000 to stop working on cancer cures and retire in Mexico".

Dr. Kendall, incidentally, reportedly died of "unknown causes" five years later, and two years after that, according to the same article, Rife "turns to alcohol, eventually needing rehabilitation".

The list of other supposed cancer cures said to have been suppressed is long enough to fill a whole book. These range from *Cannabidiol*, the little-known medical compound found in Marijuana, to a treatment that involves ingesting nothing other than regular household baking soda.

In 2009 Hollywood celebrity and cancer survivor Suzanne Somers wrote about natural cancer cures in her book *Knockout: Interviews with Doctors Who Are Curing Cancer and How To Prevent Getting it in the First Place.*

The synopsis for the book mentions that "Somers interviews doctors who are successfully using the most innovative cancer treatments—treatments that build up the body rather than tear it down."

Knockout also outlines an array of effective, alternative treatment options from doctors all over the United States. Treatments that do not involve chemotherapy or radiation and which primarily focus on building up the immune system.

The book's synopsis also mentions the "stunning testimonials from inspirational survivors using alternative treatments".

In a 2010 interview she gave on *News Max TV*, Somers spoke about her personal experience beating cancer and the wider research she conducted on alternative cures while writing *Knockout.*

"I would talk to these (alternative) doctors, interview them, and I would say to each of them 'it's all well and good for you to tell me this, but I need to talk to your patients'. They opened up their patients to me. I talked to Stage Four lung cancer, liver cancer, ovarian cancer, cervical cancer, breast cancer, prostate cancer, brain tumors – all these people living these normal, healthy lives having not been degraded by harsh chemicals. And I realized that there is another way that none of us know about."

The other way, of course, includes alternative, natural healing methods which do not involve the Medical Industrial Complex's patented (and highly profitable) chemo and radiation therapies.

To quote the natural health website *Mercola.com* once more, "There is so much you can do to lower your risk for cancer".

The site lists its "12 top cancer prevention strategies". These include:

- Food preparation – "Eat at least one-third of your food raw."

- Carbohydrates and sugar – "Reduce or eliminate processed foods, sugar/fructose and grain-based foods."

- Protein and fat – "Consider reducing your protein levels to one gram per kilogram of lean body weight."

- GMOs – "Avoid genetically engineered foods."

- Animal-based Omega-3 fats – "Normalize your ratio of Omega-3 to Omega-6 fats by taking a high-quality krill oil."

- Natural probiotics – "Optimize your gut flora…add naturally fermented food to your diet."

- Exercise – "Make regular exercise a priority…lowers insulin levels."

- Vitamin D – "*Decrease your risk of cancer by more than half* simply by optimizing your vitamin D levels with appropriate sun exposure."

- Sleep – "Make sure you are getting enough restorative sleep."

- Exposure to toxins – "Reduce your exposure to environmental toxins."

- Exposure to radiation – "Limit your exposure and protect yourself from radiation produced by cell phones, towers, base stations, and Wi-Fi stations."

- Stress management – "Stress from all causes is a major contributor to disease."

If you have cancer or know anyone who has been diagnosed with the disease, Massimo Mazzucco's 2010 documentary film *Cancer: The Forbidden Cures* is a good starting place for those searching for natural cures.

Of course, *always consult with your doctor first.* (And in case you're wondering, this is a disclaimer we had to include for legal reasons).

To be fair, the natural health sector has attracted its share of quacks, too, so *all* claims of cures should be treated with a degree of skepticism until proven. However, automatically riding roughshod over claims of natural cures, especially where those claims are supported by glowing and apparently bona-fide testimonials, is no more the answer than gullibly believing them all.

There are those who may argue that Big Pharma could also make money out of cures for cancer and that it would be a lot easier than suppressing cures. To counter that, many independent medical researchers say long-term or ongoing cancer *treatments*, like chemotherapy, would be far more profitable than delivering single-visit cures. It has been estimated that the average cancer patient spends tens of thousands of dollars on standard treatments with some even spending hundreds of thousands.

Again, Big Pharma's *repeat customers* are sick people. From a financial perspective, cured people are of little use.

As the cancer industry alone is a multi-trillion dollar industry for Big Pharma, it seems believable that if any cure was to be suppressed for financial gain it would be a cancer cure.

CHAPTER 12

Medical tests you may not need and procedures that may kill you

"Fifty percent of all doctors graduate in the bottom half of their class – Hope your surgery went well!"

–Simone Elkeles, bestselling author of Rules of Attraction

A *Reuters* report headed 'Unnecessary repeat cholesterol tests common' perhaps provides an insight into how the medical system, or machine, works.

Dated July 1, 2013, it advises that one-third of people with heart disease have their cholesterol levels checked more often than guidelines recommend, and reports that research suggests such extra testing may be a waste of time and money if it doesn't lead to improvements in patients' health.

More about those over-the-top cholesterol-level checks later in this chapter. Meantime, that *Reuters* report got us thinking…

How many medical tests and hospital procedures are unnecessary?

An exhaustive search of published medical documents, mainstream media releases and medical websites reveals the answer to that question is: far, far too many.

Even the medical profession, it seems, admits many medical procedures are unnecessary or over-used; an article dated March 5, 2013 on the well-respected *Scientific American* site states that the routine use of 130 different medical screenings, tests and treatments are often unnecessary and should be scaled back; that's according to 25 medical specialty organizations whose findings are reported on in the article.

The writer quotes a 2012 report by America's Institute of Medicine, which estimated that "in 2009 some $750 billion, or about 30 percent of all health spending, was wasted on unnecessary services and other issues, such as excessive administrative costs and fraud".

Many of the services deemed unnecessary appear on lists released by *Choosing Wisely*, an initiative of the American Board of Internal Medicine Foundation aimed at reducing needless medical interventions that waste money and can actually do more harm than good.

The *Scientific American* article reports that some of the items on the lists are familiar, giving as one example the recommendation that patients should avoid scheduling non-medically indicated labor inductions or cesarean sections before 39 weeks. It states other items are designed to reduce the use of expensive and often unnecessary imaging tests, such as early use of magnetic resonance imaging (MRI) or computed tomography scan (CT) scans for complaints that will likely go away on their own.

The report continues, "Other list items may surprise patients. The American College of Obstetricians and Gynecologists recommends that women 30 to 65 years old who are not at high risk for cervical cancer skip the annual pap smears; the research shows that conducting screenings every three years works just as well".

Professor Virginia Moyer, chair of the U.S. Preventive Services Task Force, is quoted as saying that mammography use is responsible for around one fifth of the cases of over-diagnosis of breast cancer. "Sometimes a screening leads to a false positive, after which additional tests can expose patients to unnecessary radiation or even biopsies, which carry their own risks," she says.

"Moyer points out that women have gotten mastectomies to treat small, nonaggressive cancers that were never going to affect them. 'That's a huge harm,' she says. 'Yet it can be difficult to convince people that it's okay to simply live with a cancer'."

In an article dated June 27, 2013, the *Huffington Post* lists four medical tests you may not need. Quoting a report in the *Archives of Internal Medicine*, it claims that 28% of primary care physicians admit to over-treating patients, including by ordering potentially unwarranted tests as a precaution against malpractice suits. "Unfortunately, excessive screening can open the door to unnecessary surgeries and medications -- not to mention needless anxiety".

The four tests *Huffington Post* readers are invited to reconsider (with the reporter's abridged comments in quotes) are:

- Electrocardiogram, or ECG, to detect heart abnormalities that can indicate cardiovascular disease – "There's no evidence that an ECG will reduce your risk of having a heart attack, according to…the U.S. Preventive Services Task Force".

- Upper endoscopy to diagnose conditions like gastroesophageal reflux disease – " **'You could be better off…** trying proton pump inhibitors for four to eight weeks,' says Amir Qaseem, MD, PhD, director of clinical policy at the American College of Physicians".

- Imaging (MRI, CT scans) for lower back pain to pinpoint the source of your discomfort – "MRIs not only don't improve recovery, but can increase a patient's likelihood of having surgery as much as eightfold…(and) may increase your risk for cancer".

- Bone mineral density scan to screen for osteoporosis – "If the test reveals mild bone loss, you may be prescribed osteoporosis medication, even though evidence suggests it would have little effect…**You could be better off…**waiting until you're 65 (before being screened)".

> ### *"Whenever a doctor cannot do good, he must be kept from doing harm.*
>
> *–Hippocrates*

Hospitals can also be dangerous places, according to another article the *Huffington Post* ran on April 3, 2013. Quoting the Institute of Medicine, it reports, "100,000 people die every year due to medical error -- more deaths than from car accidents, diabetes, and pneumonia. Far more patients are victims of medical error".

The report also quotes "a stunning" 2011 *Health Affairs* article in which researchers apparently discovered that medical errors occurred in one-third of all hospitalized patients. "A separate study of Medicare patients found that one in seven people in the hospital experience at least one unintended harm".

The *Huffington Post* report identifies the following as "the 10 common medical errors that can occur in the hospital": Misdiagnosis, unnecessary treatment, unnecessary tests and deadly procedures, medication mistakes, 'never events' (events that should never happen), uncoordinated care, infections (from hospital to patient), not-so-accidental 'accidents,' missed warning signs and premature discharge (from hospital).

According to the report, misdiagnosis is the most common type of medical error in a hospital; $700 billion is spent every year on unnecessary tests and treatments; medication mistakes affect 1.5 million Americans annually; 'never events' (such as scissors being left in patients' bodies) happen all too often; hospital-acquired infections, according to the Centers for Disease Control, affect 1.7 million people annually and cause nearly 100,000 deaths every year; and malfunctioning medical devices cause tens of thousands of "accidents" in hospitals every year.

Choosing Wisely, that worthy medical initiative referred to earlier, reports that "three out of four US physicians say the frequency with which doctors order unnecessary medical tests and procedures is a serious problem for America's health care system—but just as many say that the average physician orders unnecessary medical tests and procedures at least once a week".

If that admission (by US physicians) has been accurately reported – as appears to be the case given *Choosing Wisely's* impressive credentials and reputation for accuracy – then that raises alarm bells. We suspect the estimates are very conservative and the actual incidence of doctors going overboard on medical tests is even higher. Possibly much higher.

Returning to those "unnecessary repeat cholesterol tests" we touched on at the start of this chapter, *Choosing Wisely's* summation of cholesterol testing, and the statins used in those tests, is interesting. It reports that Statins are drugs that lower your cholesterol, but if you are age 75 or older and you haven't had symptoms of heart disease, "statins may be a bad idea".

The writer points out that many older adults have high cholesterol and their doctors usually prescribe statins to prevent heart disease even though, for older people, "there is no clear evidence" that high cholesterol leads to heart disease or death.

"In fact, some studies show the opposite—that older people with the lowest cholesterol levels actually have the highest risk of death…Statins can cause muscle problems, such as aches, pains, or weakness (and) may increase the risk of diabetes, cataracts, and damage to the liver, kidneys, and nerves".

This is reinforced by the *Reuters* report also referred to earlier. It quotes Dr. Michael Johansen, of the Ohio State University in Columbus, who says doctors may order more tests to meet or even exceed performance measures "and because they get paid for running a cholesterol panel".

The report refers to a US study, led by Dr. Salim Virani, of the Michael E. DeBakey Veterans Affairs Medical Center, in Houston, which tracked over 35,000 people with heart disease, and found all had their LDL ('bad') cholesterol under control even though they hadn't recently started taking any new cholesterol drugs.

"Over the 11 months after patients' most recent cholesterol test, one in three underwent a repeat test. Very few of those patients - about six percent - had any changes made to their treatment regimen as a result of the second test…People with additional health problems, such as diabetes or high blood pressure, were most likely to get their cholesterol panel repeated…The average cost of a cholesterol test is about $16…That works out to almost $204,000 in early tests in their study population - not including the cost of both patients' and doctors' time".

We haven't devoted much space in this chapter to the unseemly subject of money. (*Unseemly* in this case because certain factions in the Medical Industrial Complex are clearly creaming it financially while many of its customers/patients are struggling to pay for, or meet, the cost of their healthcare).

However, the *Reuters* report referred to above reminds us that someone is paying for every doctor's appointment, test and screening. Throw in the cost of unnecessary tests *and* repeat tests (around $16 in the case of a cholesterol test) and you begin to understand the amount of money we are talking about. It's huge!

Thankfully, as we've shown, the medical profession acknowledges there's a problem, but it will be interesting to see what the powers-that-be do about it. As per usual, we suspect it will be left to us (Joe/Jo Citizen) to keep them honest.

CHAPTER 13

Insurance – the devil's in the detail

> *"Unless you're a Warren Buffet or Bill Gates, you're one illness away from financial ruin in this country."*
>
> *–Dr. Steffie Woolhandler*

One faction we haven't devoted much space to so far is the health insurance sector – another major player in the aforementioned complex. It, too, has come in for its share of criticism. In fact, allegations of corruption have been swirling around health insurers for years.

If those unnecessary medical tests don't kill you, perhaps your medical insurance bill will!

One who intimately knows how the health insurance sector works is American Wendell Potter, a health insurance insider who shares his knowledge of the industry in a revealing article posted on the *WantToKnow.info* blog site. In it, Wendell claims he was "in a unique position to see not only how Wall Street analysts and investors influence decisions insurance company executives make but also how the industry has carried out behind-the-scenes PR and lobbying campaigns to kill or weaken any health care reform efforts that threatened insurers' profitability".

Wendell continues, "I also have seen how the industry's practices – especially those of the for-profit insurers that are under constant pressure from Wall Street to meet their profit expectations – have contributed to the tragedy of nearly 50 million people being uninsured as well as to the growing number of Americans who, because insurers now require them to pay thousands of dollars out of their own pockets before their coverage kicks in – are underinsured. An estimated 25 million of us now fall into that category.

"What I saw happening over the past few years was a steady movement away from the concept of insurance and toward 'individual responsibility,' a term used a lot by insurers and their ideological allies. This is playing out as a continuous shifting of the financial burden of health care costs away from insurers and employers and onto the backs of individuals".

Wendell concludes that rising medical bills mean fewer sick people are visiting their doctor or collecting prescriptions, and he predicts the future for many who become seriously ill will involve bankruptcy or foreclosure on their homes.

And, of course, that's exactly what's happening.

When it comes to the US medical system at least, there is no "universal healthcare" service that covers every citizen. In theory, access to cheap or else employer-sponsored private health insurance is supposed to ensure virtually everybody's covered, but what about the uninsured and the underinsured?

Call us naïve, but it seems to us that any civilized society should at least provide basic healthcare to every man, woman and child. Relying on private insurance seems like an obvious recipe for disaster. This insurance-to-fill-the-gaps approach guarantees collateral damage, including untold deaths.

Many politicians claim it would be far too expensive to provide universal healthcare, but don't blink an eye as they sign off on several trillion dollars annually on military expenditure to keep the perpetual war machine rolling. Go figure!

Let's not forget that many countries – like Japan, Australia, the UK, Sweden and New Zealand to name but a few – comfortably provide free, or at least heavily subsidized, healthcare for *all* their citizens without too much financial discomfort. So the argument from American politicians that universal healthcare would bankrupt the country just does not hold up.

This healthcare disparity between the US and the rest of the (developed) world was covered in no uncertain terms in a June 2012 article in *The Atlantic*. Headlined 'Here's a Map of the Countries That

Provide Universal Health Care (America's Still Not on It)' the article's very first line says it all. It reads, "The U.S. stands almost entirely alone among developed nations that lack universal health care."

The map referred to is a world map that highlighted those countries which provided (and still provide) free or heavily subsidized healthcare for all their citizens. Around half the world's countries were highlighted, which no doubt surprised many American readers.

The article points out that universal healthcare is available "from Europe to the Asian powerhouses to South America's southern cone to the Anglophone states of Australia, New Zealand, and Canada. The only developed outliers are a few still-troubled Balkan states, the Soviet-style autocracy of Belarus, and the U.S. of A., the richest nation in the world".

A 2013 *Real Truth* magazine article headlined 'America's Healthcare Crisis – Is There a Solution?', by Edward L. Winkfield, blames insurance for the mess that is the US healthcare system.

Winkfield highlights the exploding cost of healthcare in the last few decades. He quotes some horrifying statics, citing high medical costs being a direct cause of 60% of all bankruptcies in America and quoting a tenfold increase in healthcare expenditure in a single generation (up from $256 billion in 1980 to $2.6 trillion in 2010).

"By and large," Winkfield states, "U.S. healthcare can be summed up in one word: *insurance*. It is intended to protect individuals and families against the possibility of a devastating financial loss. Many believe this system is the only way to avoid bankruptcy and the trauma that accompanies an expensive medical bill they cannot afford to pay—in *multiple* lifetimes.

"Yet, even *with* insurance, a serious illness can lead to financial ruin".

Winkfield ends his article with a statement that basically summarizes the main theme we wish to express in this entire book:

"Those interested in *truly* resolving the healthcare dilemma *must* realize that implementing an entire system that is *proactive* – based in part on properly equipping the body to function – and not *reactive* – depending solely on medical science for a cure – is vital to solving the crisis once and for all. *This* is the factor that has been woefully missing from the healthcare equation!"

"It's sick, the price of medicine."

–The Psychedelic Furs, President Gas

Officially, 18,000 American citizens die every year for no better reason than not having an insurance card. Many have suggested that number is a very conservative estimate.

Approximately 45 million US citizens, or one American in every seven, do not have health insurance and are therefore all at risk.

Here's another statistic: besides being the number one cause in the US for bankruptcy, medical expenses are also the number one cause of homelessness.

The medical insurance system, which regularly tries to wriggle out of paying fully insured patients by using creative lawyers and loopholes buried in the fine print of contracts, is a big reason for all these horrifying statistics.

How many people have to die or suffer unnecessarily before logic *finally* sets in and everyone agrees too many citizens are falling thru the cracks in this corrupt user pays healthcare system?

It's a really perverse world where we have almost unlimited military expenditure to finance wars, where our governments readily bail out privately-owned banks with multi-trillion dollar relief packages, and yet we cannot cover the measly costs of our own citizens' basic healthcare.

People need to stop accepting the BS line that it's all just "too expensive" for governments and that less fortunate individuals must cover every single Goddamn cost by themselves. The less fortunate individuals we refer to include the mentally ill, abuse victims, war vets, the disabled, many of the elderly, the unemployed and, in many cases, employed citizens struggling to make ends meet.

As with education, you can't put a price on a population's health. It should be any government's first expenditure priority, not their last.

We will never have a civilized society until we create a fair and universal health system in which every man, woman and child – no matter their financial situation – has access to medical services when ill.

Healthcare is not a privilege, *it's a human right*.

CHAPTER 14

When did your doctor last talk to you about your diet?

"I actually like how doctors talk. I like the sound of science. I like how words you don't understand explain things you can't understand."

–American author (Ms.) R.J. Palacio

Most of you will be aware of the old adage, *You are what you eat*. It seems to us, though, that many members of the medical profession aren't aware – or, if they are, they consider it an old wives' tale.

When did your doctor last talk to you about your diet? We suspect that, more often than not, doctors only deign to discuss diet when a patient dares to raise the subject. And then, if your experience is like ours, you'll be greeted with a frosty stare or, at best, a few mumbled banalities about *not over-eating* or *the importance of a balanced diet* or *cut down on fats*.

Which leads to more (related) questions: How long do doctors-in-training spend studying nutrition at medical school? And why isn't nutrition on the curriculum alongside biochemistry, pathology, physiology and the like?

These questions and more are raised in a very appropriate discussion thread on the *ResearchGate.net* site. A random selection of comments from that thread follows:

- "We need clinicians to remember to consider nutrition when seeing/treating a patient rather than being a full nutritional expert.

However they should know basics such as basic nutritional needs and guidelines, calculating and interpreting BMI, when to give nutritional support and be aware of the importance of using nutritional screening tools to see if referral to a dietitian is required."

- "I would be a staunch supporter of making nutrition a major field of study in a medical doctors pursuit of their degree."

- "Before health care providers can get into…details about individual response to nutrients and talk about personal nutrition, they need to establish their nutrition knowledge and clinical skills foundation. For physicians this needs to happen in medical school and requires a serious effort."

- "Considering the importance of nutrition for a patient's recovery from disease and maintenance of health it is surprising that nutrition isn't a bigger part of conventional medical school education."

- "It should be within the core responsibilities of doctors to address nutrition in patient care and it is essential that all doctors know the appropriate time to make a dietitian referral."

- "Why is it so hard to understand that robust familiarity with nutrition is equally or even more important (than surgery training)?"

To add some balance to the discussion, one contributor (from the University of Jordan) to the above thread observes that nutrition is "a specialized field and huge in its content." He adds, "Medical students (are) overwhelmed by texts, labs, and courses. It requires an evolutionary plan to incorporate nutrition with medicine curricula".

Medical educators at least pay lip service to the importance of nutrition, and they appear to be in general agreement that there's not enough instruction on this topic in today's medical schools.

For example, the American Academy of Family Physicians (AAFP) addresses this via its official online site *AAFP News*. In an article dated May 17, 2010, the writer reports that although most medical schools (in the US) offer some form of nutrition education, only one-quarter require a dedicated nutrition course.

The article continues, "In fact, the amount of nutrition education that medical students receive is so 'inadequate' that 'medical school graduates feel unprepared to intervene in their patients' care with regard to nutrition,' according to the UNC preliminary survey results".

Another 2010 report – this one published by the US National Library of Medicine in conjunction with the National Institutes of Health – concludes that "The amount of nutrition education that medical students receive continues to be inadequate".

That report summarizes a survey of 109 medical schools, which revealed that "most (103) required some form of nutrition education" of their students. The most disturbing revelation, however, is that "Overall, medical students received 19.6 contact hours of nutrition instruction during their medical school careers".

19.6 contact hours of nutrition instruction? During a med school course that takes, what, four or five years at least?

"The downside to becoming a doctor, I think, is it's a very long process; four years of medical school, three years of internship, two years of residency, umpteen years of specialization, and then finally you get to be what you have trained almost all your life for."

—South Korean artist Jim Lee

Let's face it, sensible eating is probably the best single thing we can do to help ensure a healthy future as food governs the functions of our organs and figures prominently in both the contracting of illness and disease, and in our recovery from those ailments.

The link between diet and health is well proven and, more importantly, widely acknowledged by doctors, for ailments such as diabetes and heart disease, but are roundly ignored by them in treating other human conditions – cancer being one of those. Indeed, mainstream (Western) medicine seems to go out of its way to discourage cancer patients from making too much of the cancer-diet connection.

The good health site *HoneyColony.com* neatly addresses this in an article quoting Dr. Carolyn Dean, a medical advisory board member of the nonprofit Nutritional Magnesium Association. She says, "There are many reasons why diet is not stressed in cancer treatment" and "Most of them stem from the fact that medicine does not put any emphasis on nutrition in medical school...In about 3,500 hours of typical medical school training, maybe one, two, or three hours' worth of classes are devoted to basic nutrition".

So now it's only three hours of basic nutrition at most...in a five-year course! Lordy.

The cancer-diet connection is also examined by the *BBC* online in an article dated May 19, 2013. Presenter Sheila Dillon, herself a cancer patient, observes, "Thousands of scientific papers have been published on the link between diet and the treatment and prevention of cancer, but in practice food is still considered a marginal aspect of cancer care".

Ms Dillon continues, "Research confirmed that in most cancer centres in the UK, diet is still seen as almost meaningless in cancer treatment and aftercare. Yet there is good science available on the subject, though not a lot of it is what medics call 'gold standard' science.

"There are almost no double-blinded, large scale, studies done on people because they are expensive, very hard to do and there is no financial incentive. Who would make serious profit out of the discovery that mushrooms kill cancer cells?

"Most of the research has been done on cancer cells in the laboratory or on animals. What the best of it shows is interesting implications in a range of foods.

"One of the best-researched foods (in the US and Ireland) is the spice turmeric. Curcumin is a chemical compound found in the root of turmeric, which has a general anti-inflammatory effect and quite specific effects on several forms of cancer, including mine," she says.

"Research has also been conducted on berries containing ellagic acid, which seems to curb cancer cells' ability to grow their own blood supply, mushrooms (the polysaccharides), green tea, as well as the cabbage and onion families.

Ms Dillon concludes, "From my experience as a cancer patient I think many people fear that they are being ungrateful for the medical care they have had by bringing up issues such as diet".

Still in the UK, if a report published by the British Psychological Society is correct, "too many people with eating disorders are being dismissed by doctors as simply having peculiar habits with food".

The report, dated February 25, 2014, is based on the findings of *Cosmopolitan UK* magazine and the charity Beat which warned that "around 1.6 million people currently have an eating disorder in Britain, half of whom have being diagnosed with an EDNOS (eating disorder not otherwise specified) that is separate from anorexia or bulimia".

The article continues, "However, many of these patients could be left waiting up to two years for treatment in the form of cognitive behavioural therapy because GPs do not view their symptoms as sufficiently serious to warrant urgent investigation".

By now it should be clear there's a serious disconnect between (most) doctors and the role of nutrition in their patients' health. Whether you blame those who set the already crowded curricula at medical schools or whether you blame the tunnel vision mainstream medicine has regarding diet, the fact remains there's a problem. And in many independent medical researchers eye it's a *big problemo*.

> *"First the doctor told me the good news: I was going to have a disease named after me."*
>
> *–Steve Martin*

Of course, good nutrition and healthy diets have been compromised by the advent of GMO's, or genetically modified organisms. To cite Wikipedia, "A GMO is any organism whose genetic material has been altered using genetic engineering techniques. GMOs are the source of genetically modified foods and are also widely used in scientific research and to produce goods other than food".

Now we can't blame the Medical Industrial Complex for the advent of genetically modified foods, but there are some parallels as you'll see. For the sake of this little exercise, replace the term *Big Pharma* with the equally emotive term *Big Brother* and you'll get the picture.

Genetic modification has been around, in its modern form, since the 1970's – and has sparked a major debate ever since. Advocacy groups and opponents of GMO have long claimed that genetically modified food presents potential dangers to the very future of Mankind's health.

The debate is no less fierce amongst members of our 'Underground

Knowledge' discussion group on *Goodreads.com*. It was prompted by one member who asked, "What's the deal with GMO's? Why are they banned in Europe and not in the USA? If there is nothing wrong with them then why is the government NOT requiring that food be labeled as containing GMOed items? Why is Monsanto so adamant that labeling NOT be required or permitted? Who are these people anyway? It should be my decision as to what I put in my body!"

Random samples of members' responses follow. (Names withheld):

- "Yep, the whole GM thing is scary- just like tales of chemtrails or tap water poisoning us- but, yeah, we should be able to know the truth about what GM products are in what foods, and I've read stuff before about even with labels, there can still sometimes be a GM product 'through a loop hole'."

- "It's a worrying state of affairs when we don't know if our meat is cow or horse, and we're digesting more and more GM products, and there never seems to be any straight answers as to who to trust with these kinds of subjects."

- "Food should just be food! Why did 'they' have to go mess with nature? If they could restructure the air and make a buck out of it, they would!"

- "My wife and I have stopped eating anything processed and only eat organic as much as possible."

- "I saw an interesting program on TV this morning. They were talking about fortified breakfast cereal. The man ground up some of the flakes and mixed it with some liquid in a breaker and dropped in a magnetic stirrer. After a few moments he removed the stirrer and gently rinsed it off. Guess what was all over it? Iron filings! Apparently they are supposed to be in the cereal."

You may be asking what genetically modified foods have to do with medicine. Well, technically speaking, not much. However, the point is if some of the food supply has been poisoned or otherwise become toxic and therefore is partially responsible for the dramatic recent increases of certain diseases (such as autoimmune disorders), then surely doctors would be amongst those who'd recognize this fact. But is that a fair assumption given most doctors do not seem to commonly believe what we put into our bodies matters that much?

Returning to our original question – When did your doctor last talk to you about your diet? If the answer to that is *Never*, perhaps it's time you did. Talk to him/her, that is. Be it to address high cholesterol, an excess weight problem, a heart condition, cancer or high blood pressure, perhaps it's time to have that little chat.

If doctors are aware their patients are diet-conscious *and* if they're constantly reminded nutrition is important to them, perhaps they'll fall into line and give it (nutrition) the importance it deserves when it comes to treating people.

Hopefully, this chapter has provided you with some ammunition to fire their way.

We must add a little footnote here and acknowledge that the inference that doctors are not nutrition-minded or, for that matter, not supportive of alternative health measures is very much a generalization; we are aware there's a growing number of physicians (and other health providers) in mainstream medicine who are very knowledgeable about nutrition and alternative health, and who incorporate this knowledge into their everyday practice.

Unfortunately, they are very much in the minority.

Chapter 15

The alternative health sector – warts and all

There's no doubt the terms *Medical Industrial Complex, Big Pharma, prescription drugs, doctors' kickbacks, medical fraud* and *suppressed curves* are emotive terms – as are the terms *alternative health, natural health, alternative treatments, natural cures* and *health supplements*. And the battle lines for each are well established.

Though the lines between mainstream medicine and alternative health are often blurred, and confusion reigns in some areas, most people lean toward one or the other for the management of their health.

Increasingly, however, growing numbers of people are looking to utilize the best of both. Critics of mainstream medicine have been quick to seize on this, pointing out that the willingness of more and more people to embrace alternative health worldwide equates to huge financial losses for the Medical Industrial Establishment.

Among the strategies some of those same critics employ to attract new followers is to trot out a myriad of conspiracy theories – some more conspiracy fact than theory, but many a combination of distortions of the truth, half-truths and flat-out fabrications.

Wikipedia provides the following insight into some of these medical conspiracies:

Conspiracy theories, false claims, fraud and greed aren't the sole domain of the Medical Industrial Complex. The alternative health sector or the natural health industry, whichever your preference, is also a very lucrative industry that has, as we discovered, attracted its share of controversy – some of it deserved.

Just as Big Pharma and the other major players in the Medical Industrial Complex have attracted their share of criticism – some would say more than their share – so, too, has the alternative health sector. And in many ways alternative medicine and mainstream medicine are not mutually exclusive and tend to overlap.

And that overlapping aspect means that, perhaps paradoxically, the alternative health sector is at least partially within the Medical Industrial Complex.

To recap on this sector, *alternative health* encompasses dietary supplements, natural and alternative (or complementary) medicines, plus therapies and treatments ranging from well-known modalities like massage therapy, acupuncture, homeopathy and naturopathy to more exotic and lesser known ones such as chelation therapy, ear candling and moxibustion.

The alternative health sector is vast, is growing rapidly and, like the Medical Industrial Complex, is mighty profitable. Not as profitable as Big Pharma perhaps, but nevertheless highly commercial and lucrative.

And with that profitability come problems. Naturally. (Excuse the pun).

Firstly, we examine mainstream medicine's stance on alternative medicine. It's pretty obvious most doctors would prefer the *alternative* crowd go away or, better still, keep quiet. After all, more and more consumers are turning away from mainstream medicine to embrace or at least try alternatives, so jobs and profits are on the line.

Doctors are quick to point out the dangers of some dietary supplements and alternative medicines – and with some justification. Any Joe/Jo Citizen can call him or herself an alternative health practitioner and/or open a health shop dispensing supplements to an unwary and unsuspecting public.

The American Cancer Society (ACS) addresses this very point, advising that the FDA requires zero proof that dietary supplements have been tested before they are sold even though those dispensing the supplements are allowed to make certain health claims.

On its website, the ACS points out that dietary supplements are handled by the FDA in just the opposite way to medicines. "For example, drugs, even ones that are sold over the counter, must be carefully tested to find out about their risks and side effects before they can be sold. They also must be proven effective".

The ACS acknowledges there are new requirements in place regarding how dietary supplements must be made and labeled, but points out no-one requires that they be tested to find out whether they actually help. And, it states, most dietary supplements are generally regarded as safe by the FDA until proven otherwise – meaning that dietary supplements can be sold without proving anything. In other words, the burden of proof is on the FDA to show that it isn't safe.

ACS says this is very different from mainstream drugs. "With medicines, the maker of the drug must show that it works and it's safe – before they can ever sell it".

The article continues, "One of the reasons for these differences is that, unlike drugs, supplements are not intended to treat, diagnose, prevent, or cure diseases. This means supplements should not make claims such as 'reduces arthritic pain' or 'treats heart disease.' Claims like these can only be made for drugs that have been proven to do what they claim. Products that are proven to have a significant effect on any disease are considered drugs by the FDA and are strictly regulated.

"Other methods, such as, acupuncture, and naturopathy have come into wide use with no requirement for testing to see how well they work…Of course, regulations, licenses, or certificates do not guarantee safe and effective treatment from any provider, but they can give you information and may offer more options if something does go wrong".

Scan back issues of any metropolitan newspaper or conduct a quick search online and you'll find numerous accounts of bogus health supplements, fake natural cures and the like.

The UK's *Daily Mail* ran a damning article headed 'Alternative cures are bogus'. It quotes Exeter University's Professor Edzard Ernst as saying some therapies are positively dangerous, but desperate patients are misled into using them instead of conventional treatments which have the backing of medical research.

Professor Ernst, who is introduced as "the nation's only professor of complementary medicine," also asserts that cancer patients are being duped by "criminal and fraudulent" claims that alternative therapies can cure their disease. He describes such claims as lies that are costing lives. And he says, "In terms of treatment and prolongation of life, not only is the use of alternative and complementary medicine not supported by data, it is very often fraudulent and even criminal. It can be quite dangerous from the patient's point of view. Many give up conventional treatment and this predictably leads to disaster".

The article reports that increasing numbers of cancer patients are turning to complementary therapies – many of them found on the Internet, ranging from herbal remedies to acupuncture. "(Professor Ernst) said there are half a million Internet sites promoting complementary therapies for cancer. The 'cures' were all bogus, he said".

In the same article, Dr Eric Winer, associate professor of medicine at Harvard University, is quoted as saying not a single cancer patient had been cured by complementary therapy. "He said ingested therapies posed the most serious threat as they can interfere with orthodox treatment".

Of course this is one doctor's viewpoint and an extreme viewpoint in our opinion.

Professor Ernst is even more vociferous than Dr. Winer on the *Better Health* website, which he contributes to. In a post dated July 7, 2014, he accuses "pseudo-scientists" of "creating medical research to support bogus therapies".

The professor expresses some relief that "today there finally seems to be a consensus that alternative medicine can and should be submitted to scientific tests much like any other branch of health care".

Incidentally, his understanding of the term *pseudo-scientist* is: "It describes a person who thinks he/she knows the truth about his/her subject well before he/she has done the actual research. A pseudo-scientist is keen to understand the rules of science in order to corrupt science; he/she aims at using the tools of science not to test his/her assumptions and hypotheses, but to prove that his/her preconceived ideas were correct".

In this particular post, Professor Ernst outlines, somewhat tongue in cheek, nine steps to follow to become a top pseudo-scientist. If nothing else it makes for an entertaining read – Step 8 (**"Play with statistics until you get the desired result"**) being a case in point.

So there you have it: critical examples and reports – real or imagined, depending on which side of the fence you sit – of the state of the alternative health sector and some of the problems that apparently pervade it.

There are many more examples and case studies we could cite – enough to fill this book in fact. However, the message should be clear by now. The message is that, globally, there are big profits to be made in alternative health and, as is the case in any lucrative field, where big bucks are on offer corruption and shady practices are never far away.

Equally, in the healthcare sector generally, it should now be clear that corruption isn't the sole domain of Big Pharma.

CHAPTER 16

Human guinea pigs

*Like all companies in the legal drug trade,
KaizerSimonsKovak needed to test new drugs before
releasing them onto the market. While its competitors
tested their new drugs mostly on rats, mice and
monkeys, KSK had the advantage of being able to test
them on humans. No KSK employee, or indeed anyone
outside Omega, was aware of that, however. All testing
was contracted out – to another Omega-owned
company. And its modus operandi was far from legal.*

–The Orphan Uprising

On May 14, 2013, German news magazine Der Spiegel ran an article about international drug companies conducting illegal tests on impoverished citizens in India. The article stated, "The practice is forbidden, but the use of subcontractors makes it difficult to detect".

In 2008, it was revealed that over a two-and-a- half-year period of testing medicines at the All India Institute of Medical Sciences (AIIMS), 49 babies had died during clinical studies. *The Times of India* reported this incident in no uncertain terms in an August 19, 2008 article headlined *49 babies die during clinical trials at AIIMS*.

Such experimentation is in direct violation of the World Medical Association's *Declaration of Helsinki*, which requires subjects in tests to be shielded from harm. However, in the AIIMS scandal the accused international drug manufacturers denied all responsibility for, or even any involvement in, the tests on the babies.

Besides India, it's common for Big Pharma to carry out illegal testing of medicines and drugs on human subjects in Russia, Brazil and China.

So maybe bestselling author and former lawyer John Grisham's inclusion of a corrupt US pharmaceutical conglomerate illegally testing dangerous drugs on unwitting volunteers – some as young as 14 – in Africa in his (excellent) novel *The Litigators* is not totally fictitious or far-fetched.

> *"It is no measure of health to be well adjusted to a profoundly sick society."*
>
> *–Jiddu Krishnamurti*

Africa has long been used for dubious clinical trials of new drugs by Big Pharma – something that concerns human rights activists and ethical watchdogs, but whose concerns seem only to fall on deaf ears. (What is it about Africa that Western governments and *Big Business* seem to think can be so abused)?

The litany of abuses by pharmaceutical companies against citizens of African countries seems to go on forever. Random examples of just a few of these abuses follow:

BBC News reported on June 5, 2007, that Nigeria filed charges against the pharmaceutical company Pfizer, accusing it of carrying out improper trials for an anti-meningitis drug. The report states, "The government is seeking $7bn (£3.5bn) in damages for the families of children who allegedly died or suffered side-effects after being given Trovan".

The report continues, "Pfizer - the world's largest pharmaceutical company - tested the experimental antibiotic Trovan in Kano during an outbreak of meningitis which had affected thousands in 1996. Some 200 children were tested. Pfizer say 11 of them died of meningitis, but Kano officials say about 50 died whilst others developed mental and physical deformities".

The *BBC News* report concludes, "This is the first time Nigeria's federal government has filed charges against Pfizer but individual families have previously taken legal action. The separate case in Kano - in which the state is seeking $2.7bn in compensation - has been running for more than two years".

Some of you will recall the blockbuster film *The Constant Gardener* (based on the bestselling book of the same name) revolved around clinical trials in African slums. What you may not know, however, is the story was inspired by the true-life meningitis travesty described above.

Many critics argue it's no accident that the big drug companies do much of their drug testing on impoverished Third World subjects. There's less publicity, less legal liability, less financial risk, less fallout.

A Green Road Project observes on its *agreenroad* blog site that many African nations cannot afford to offer medicine for their citizens without subsidies from multinational pharmaceutical corporations.

The *Green Road* editorial states: "To court these pharmaceutical corporations, some African nations minimize legal regulations on the conduct of medical research, which prevents potential legal battles from arising. This forces some Africans to make a Hobson's choice: 'experimental medicine or no medicine at all.' People living in the rural or slum area are also more vulnerable to experimentation because they are more likely to be illiterate and to misunderstand the effects of the experimentation".

And Wikipedia catalogues the incidence of improper HIV/AIDS trials conducted by US physicians and University of Zimbabwe personnel on HIV-positive African subjects in the mid-1990's. The entry reads: "It included testing of over 17,000 women for a medication that prevents mother-to-child transmission of HIV/AIDS...Half of these women received a placebo that has no effect, making transmission likely. As a result, an estimated 1000 babies contracted HIV/AIDS although a proven life-saving regimen already existed".

Human guinea pigs are nothing new of course. In America early last century, Indiana passed the world's first eugenics-motivated sterilization law. (Eugenics, also referred to as *social engineering*, being the science of improving a population by controlled breeding to increase the occurrence of desirable heritable characteristics). Thirty US states soon followed Indiana's lead by making it legal to sterilize those deemed genetically inferior, especially psychiatric patients.

Those with certain types of mental illness weren't the only ones sterilized en masse, however. Promiscuous women, prostitutes and females with perceived negative sexual orientations like bisexuality or lesbianism were often sterilized by authorities, while for men sterilizations were regularly done to curb excessive aggression in certain types of criminals.

Outside the US, various countries including Brazil, Belgium, Sweden and Canada implemented the policy of sterilizing citizens ruled not worthy of reproduction.

Genocide. Sterilization of the mentally ill, blacks, homosexuals and other *undesirables*. Euthenasia. Forced pregnancies and birth control. Racial segregation. Compulsory abortions. Genetic screening. These are examples of eugenics practices and policies adopted to varying degrees by various countries until commonsense prevailed and *most* countries banned such practices.

During the years that eugenics legislation was in effect in the US, around 65,000 American citizens were used as human guinea pigs and forcibly sterilized. Although compulsory sterilization has been considered a human rights violation in most parts of America since WW2, the laws were not overturned in many states until decades later. Virginia, for example, did not overturn its sterilization law until 1974.

From 1932 until 1972, the US Public Health Service deceptively conducted a clinical study known as the *Tuskegee Syphilis Experiment*. The notorious study was designed to monitor the progression of syphilis in African-American men who were led to believe they were receiving free treatment from the Government for the sexually transmitted disease. The infamous 40-year experiment involved medical professionals surreptitiously refusing treatment to black patients infected with syphilis.

Revelations by whistleblowers of the Tuskegee syphilis experiment led to US law changes concerning patient protection and informed consent for medical studies.

Now here's an experiment that defies belief. It involved the proven and acknowledged infection of Guatemalan orphans, schoolchildren, psychiatric patients, prison inmates and many others with venereal diseases in the late 1940's by – wait for it – American public health doctors!

Through the late Nineties and early 2000's rumors of deliberate infection of Guatemalans became whispers until finally, in 2005, hard evidence of what one senior US health official described as "a dark chapter in the history of medicine" was produced.

The world learned that for years American public health doctors deliberately infected hundreds of Guatemalans with syphilis and other venereal diseases. Apparently, the reason for this was to test the effectiveness of penicillin on those infections.

International Rights Advocates claim more than 5000 Guatemalans were experimented on and, in the course of those experiments, over 1000 were infected with venereal diseases.

One experiment entailed syphilis-infected prostitutes sleeping with prisoners in Guatemalan prisons. It transpires that prisoners not infected were administered the bacteria by injection or other means. While those who contracted syphilis were given antibiotics, it remains unclear exactly how many – if any – were cured.

The experiments, funded by America's National Institutes of Health, were facilitated by Guatemalan health officials without the informed consent of subjects. Reports show at least 80 deaths resulted – with some estimates being much higher.

In October 2010 the US Government officially apologized for the actions of American citizens involved in the whole ugly business.

In a joint statement, Secretary of State Hillary Rodham Clinton and Health and Human Services Secretary Kathleen Sebelius said, "Although these events occurred more than 64 years ago, we are outraged that such reprehensible research could have occurred under the guise of public health. We deeply regret that it happened, and we apologize to all the individuals who were affected by such abhorrent research practices."

In a twist to the revelation, the New York Times issue of October 1, 2010 reported – beneath the banner headline *U.S. apologizes for syphilis tests in Guatemala* – that "The public health doctor who led the experiment, John C. Cutler, would later have an important role in the Tuskegee study".

The study referred to was the US Public Health Service's unethical and infamous Tuskegee syphilis experiment that saw African-American males with syphilis deliberately left untreated for 40 years (from 1932 to 1972). But that's a whole other story.

Getting back to the Guatemala experiments, a (US) Presidential Commission for the Study of Bioethical Issues concluded that, after an intensive nine-month investigation, "The Guatemala experiments involved gross violations of ethics…It is the Commission's firm belief that many of the actions undertaken in Guatemala were especially

117

egregious moral wrongs because many of the individuals involved held positions of public institutional responsibility."

Our research into this experiment has not uncovered reports of successful prosecutions against any of the American health officials or medical staffers involved in this travesty. Nor has it revealed whether any of the experiment's subjects have received compensation for the atrocities committed. We can only assume the answer is *No* to both those questions.

Returning to the aforementioned article in the German news magazine *Der Spiegel* and to the present-day activities of drug companies, "Several studies indicate that more than half of all drug trials worldwide take place in newly industrialized countries. Not only are the studies cheaper to carry out there, but many participants are thankful that they are being cared for in any way at all. The companies are lured by the prospect that established international standards are less stringently applied than they are in Western Europe, Japan or the United States."

It strikes us that more human guinea pigs will be abused and more deaths will occur until something changes either in the morality of the Medical Industrial Complex itself (don't hold your breath!) or else in international regulatory bodies and watchdog organizations.

CONNECTING THE DOTS...

Human guinea pigs / Medical fraud / Political ambitions superseding the health of the people / Suppressing cancer cures / Health insurers screwing customers / Toxic immunizations for children / Big Pharma making money at all costs / Hospital misadventures / Doctors receiving kickbacks / Overprescribing of prescription drugs / Sinking natural health products in a sea of red tape etc. etc.

It's obvious something has run amuck in the medical field. What should be the noblest profession has been severely compromised by the various conflicting interests we have highlighted in the preceding pages, including rampant commercialism, political selfishness and dogmatic academia.

Having now reached the end of this book, we hope you won't be so willing in future to entrust medical professionals with decision-making responsibility concerning *your* health. Next time your doctor tells you that prescribed medication has no side-effects, we expect you'll be doing some research of your own or at least getting a second opinion.

It's our belief that taking back control of your health is essentially a self-respect issue: you are broadcasting the message that "My body belongs to me and I get the final say as to what goes into it and what doesn't".

Despite all the gloom and doom, as we said from the outset, there are many honorable people within the medical establishment who are doing incredible things for their fellow Man. Of that there is no doubt. So in the end it's not about pointing fingers, but collectively *demanding* the fairest healthcare services for *all* citizens: young and old, rich and poor.

Given there is little to no quality of life without your health, perhaps there's no more important issue facing the planet right now than providing decent healthcare for everyone.

Is it a complex dilemma to resolve? Yes.

Is it impossible? No.

THE END

If you liked this book, the authors would greatly appreciate a review from you on Amazon.

If you wish to discuss more about the material in this book, or other interrelated 'alternative' topics, we invite you to join our Underground Knowledge discussion group on Goodreads.com

An excerpt from *Genius Intelligence*, book one in *The Underground Knowledge Series*, follows…

GENIUS
INTELLIGENCE:

Secret Techniques and Technologies to Increase IQ

THE UNDERGROUND KNOWLEDGE SERIES

**James & Lance
MORCAN**

CONTENTS

FOREWORD

This book is part of *The Underground Knowledge Series*, written by James & Lance Morcan, authors of a much needed, perceptive summary of the darker aspects of world reality titled *The Orphan Conspiracies*, which I also wrote a foreword for.

I was employed for many years as a senior research scientist developing naval underwater weapon systems at the Technical Research and Development Institute of the Ministry of Defense, Japan. During this period, I spent a lot of time in my private life studying *Number Theory*, which is a branch of pure mathematics devoted primarily to the study of the integers, or whole numbers.

From this mathematical research, I came across the enigma of Srinivasa Ramanujan (Figure 1), an Indian genius mathematician who, with almost no formal training, discovered many complex formulas and made extraordinary contributions to mathematical analysis and number theory. Ramanujan often said the Goddess of Namakkal inspired him with formulae at night while he was dreaming and that each morning, upon awakening, he would write down the results of these vivid dreams.

For many years, I could not understand the mental processes that lead to Ramanujan's advanced mathematical findings. However, after studying the human brain from the standpoint of superluminal particles, I eventually came to the conclusion that everyone's brain has the potential to connect to an outer field of consciousness, which has also been termed by more mystical thinkers as the Universal Mind.

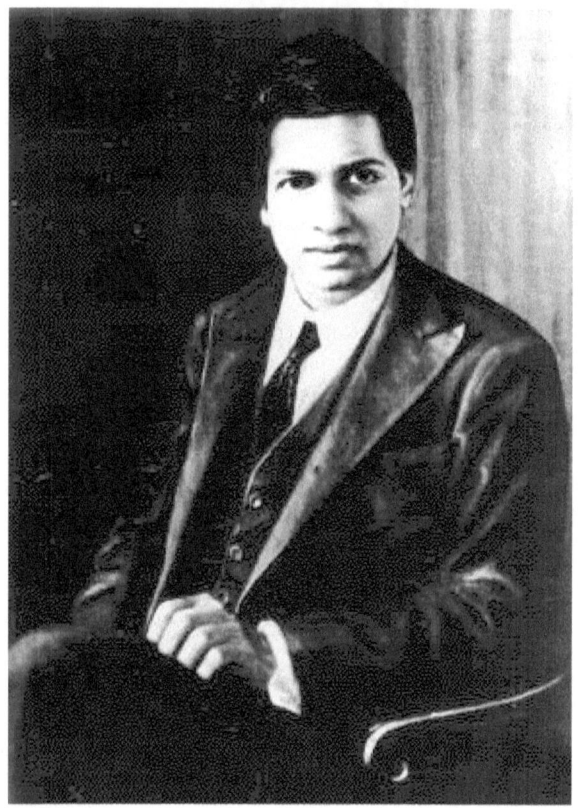

Figure 1: Srinivasa Ramanujan

To summarize my research on the brain, I wrote *Superluminal Particles and Hypercomputation*, which was published by LAMBERT Academic Publishing in early 2014. Soon after its publication, I was contacted by James Morcan, one of the authors of *Genius Intelligence*, who felt that my theories on superluminal particles could support his and Lance Morcan's suppositions about the nature of genius.

This book you are now reading contains a wide range of genius methods – all of which have the potential to increase your IQ. You'll read about everything from speed reading to brain gland activation to sleep learning to smart drugs to virtual reality training.

I believe this is a much needed book for those who sense there are faster and easier ways to learn and study than the methods currently being taught in mainstream education systems.

Lastly, I sincerely hope that the publication of *Genius Intelligence* contributes to a global awakening to assist us to hold enough truth in our minds to change this world for better.

Dr. Takaaki Musha

Director of the Advanced-Science Technology Research Organization, Yokohama, Japan.

Former senior research scientist at the Technical Research and Development Institute of the Ministry of Defense, Japan.

INTRODUCTION

The genesis for this book was fiction rather than reality.

Now we've revealed that, you would be forgiven for assuming none of what follows on the mightily complex subject of intelligence and increasing IQ is true.

Before we attempt to put your mind at ease on that score, we have a few more revelations to get out of the way...

Neither of us has any formal education qualifications of note, having barely completed high school. Nor has either of us ever taken an IQ test and therefore it cannot be proven we have high intelligence just as it cannot be disproven we are complete idiots!

About now, you'd also be forgiven for asking why we, of all people, have written a book on intelligence and the nature of genius.

On the fiction versus reality issue, it's not quite as alarming as it sounds, we hope.

You see, the fictional reference actually relates to our international thriller series of novels titled *The Orphan Trilogy*.

The decision to write this thriller series was made a decade ago, and it marks the commencement of our journey. A journey to discover what makes a genius and, more importantly, what makes a genius tick.

In *The Ninth Orphan*, book one in the trilogy, our mysterious lead character (who is known only as Nine) is not only an assassin, but also a mental genius who exhibits a level of intelligence rarely if ever seen in any character in literature. Nine has a photographic memory, can read entire books in five minutes flat and speaks dozens of languages.

Plus he learns new skills extremely fast and is highly adaptable – so much so he's nicknamed *the human chameleon.*

How Nine reached that level of intelligence, though, is merely implied or hinted at in the first book in the series.

In its prequel, *The Orphan Factory*, we had to design an education system that would reveal exactly how Nine and his fellow orphans grew up to become that smart. This was quite a challenge as our setting was no Ivy League college. Rather, it was the Pedemont Orphanage, a rundown institution in Riverdale, one of Chicago's poorest neighborhoods.

Having both gone through the traditional education system and finding it laborious and uninspiring, we quickly discovered it was fun to brainstorm alternative and more advanced forms of study for our trilogy. Even so, it took many years of investigating accelerated learning methods – some rare, some not so rare – before we felt confident enough to write about what it would take to create youngsters with intellects as advanced as those of our Pedemont orphans.

All the insights unearthed during that 10-year investigative period (spent examining the great historical minds and studying little-known intelligence boosting methods) are revealed in *Genius Intelligence.*

Highlights of our exploration into the world of super learning include many fascinating discoveries, which were totally new – to us at least and, we expect, in most cases will be new to you, too – and which were certainly outside our personal experience collectively and individually.

Those discoveries include:

- Individuals (living and dead) with IQ's far higher than Einstein's.

- Brain waves common to geniuses – and the various ways to induce those brain waves.

- Mental techniques the world's elite and A-List celebrities are quietly using to help them process information while they're asleep or in *virtual* worlds.

- Chemical substances students and academics the world over employ to kick-start the brain into overdrive.

- Cutting-edge technologies business tycoons and professional athletes employ to achieve a mental edge on their competitors.

Beyond these random examples, one of the key discoveries we made is that every human brain has enormous potential – possibly even *unlimited* potential.

No matter the challenging circumstances – whether ADHD, dyslexia or mental illness – it makes no difference when it comes to the brain's *latent* potential. The capacity for achieving genius levels of intelligence remains the same. After all, there has been many a genius with learning disabilities, hyperactivity and genetic brain disorders.

The latest scientific studies have revealed extraordinary findings. The brain is much more flexible and adaptable than previously thought. It can evolve and creatively work around limitations and nullify them.

Examples of this phenomenon even include brain-damaged individuals who have been shown to be capable of achieving equal intelligence to the average person.

How or why this is possible is because of the brain's incredible capacity to restructure itself.

This rewiring process falls under a category in neuroscience known as *neuroplasticity* – a broad term used to describe the brain's ability to form new neural connections or to reorganize itself in an attempt to overcome or diminish the effects of old age, substance abuse or traumatic head injury.

Neuroplasticity is scientific proof that intelligence is *not* something that is locked by a certain age or that cannot fluctuate or increase.

Not receiving a college degree or even a high school education doesn't mean genius abilities are out of the question. The same applies for those who come from a background of extreme poverty.

History is littered with examples of uneducated and semi-educated individuals from impoverished backgrounds who have gone on to educate themselves and deliver revolutionary breakthroughs within academic circles, the corporate world, the arts and other walks of life.

When the brain's potential is fully unleashed, there can be few if any limitations (Figure 2). Anyone who tells you otherwise isn't up-to-date with the latest scientific findings on the brain and is exhibiting their ignorance. For the brain's potential *is* the human potential…

The other crucial discovery – perhaps *the* most crucial – to come out of our research is that higher intelligence is not necessarily something you're born with or genetically predisposed toward. In fact, most instances of above-the-ordinary intelligences are usually *acquired* thru superior learning techniques – many of which we cover in detail in this book.

Reading about the greatest minds in history, including recent history, more often than not reveals the individuals concerned (or people close to them) employed specific learning methods. The examples we cite throughout this book shatter the myth that geniuses are always born with exceptional intelligence and/or talent.

Certainly, there are those born with amazing abilities not fostered by educational methods, but our research has revealed these naturally gifted geniuses are definitely the exception, not the norm.

A classic example of this natural born genius myth is Wolfgang Amadeus Mozart (Figure 3) whom most believe was simply a wunderkind, or virtuoso, from infancy. Many brain researchers have also described the Austrian composer as someone who just had incredible musical and artistic abilities from birth.

However, as with most geniuses, there is a significant body of evidence to support the contentious theory that Mozart's brilliance was as much the result of *nurture* as it was *nature*, if not more so.

It is true the musical prodigy was composing by five, and by seven or so he was performing for audiences throughout Europe. And while achievements like that, at those early ages, are certainly extraordinary, the key point is that Mozart came from a musical family and was pushed to excel musically. As soon as he could walk and talk, in fact, or even earlier if you stop to consider he was exposed to classical compositions while still in his mother's womb.

The young Mozart's father Leopold was a renowned composer in his own right and an ambitious musical teacher who wanted his son to achieve greatness. History tells us that Leopold forced Mozart Junior to practice for many hours a day even before he had reached school age.

It has been estimated that by the time Mozart was six he had already spent about 4000 hours studying music.

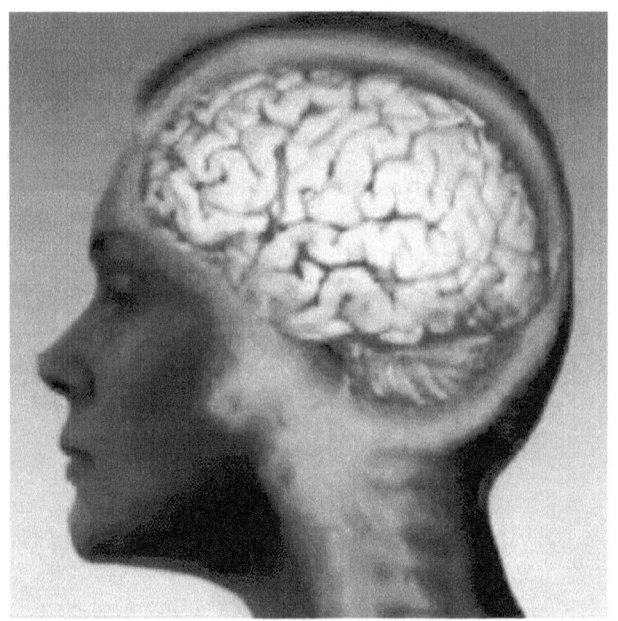

Figure 2: *Above: The brain...unlimited potential?*

"Human brain female side view"
by National Institute of Health

Licensed under Public Domain via Wikimedia Commons

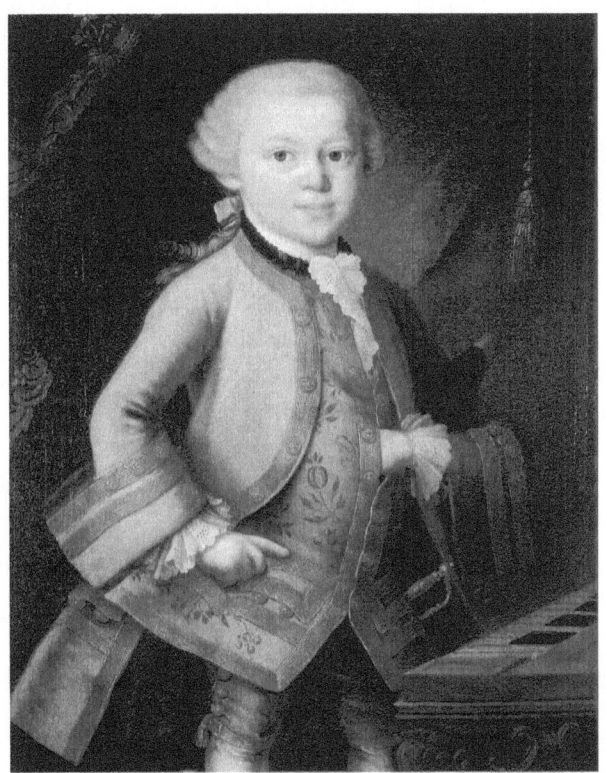

Figure 3: *Mozart as a child*

"Wolfgang-amadeus-mozart 2" by Anonymous possibly by Pietro
Antonio Lorenzoni (1721-1782)
Portrait owned by the Mozarteum, Salzburg.
Licensed under Public Domain via Wikimedia Commons

Perhaps a modern-day equivalent to Mozart's father would be someone like Richard Williams, father of legendary American tennis champions Serena and Venus Williams. Upon deciding tennis was the way out of the 'ghetto', Williams Sr. pushed his daughters day after day from a young age in his relentless quest for them to become world champions.

Classical music experts have noted that many of Mozart's childhood compositions are mostly rearrangements of other (older) composers' works. Not being experts in classical music – or any music for that matter – we can't comment, but if true that would further undermine the enduring myth about the great composer being an innate genius who could rely solely on his natural talent and who hardly needed to practice.

We found that nine out of ten biographies of geniuses reveal forgotten or previously unmentioned examples of intelligence-enhancing techniques and/or technologies these individuals employed on their path to greatness.

Traditionally, IQ has been perceived as a genetic trait in much the same way an individual's height or body type is perceived – in other words a fixed trait, or state, and therefore (thought to be) something that could never be altered.

In recent years, however, there has been an explosion of new scientific studies, which make a mockery of that assumption. These show that cognitive training, whether by mental techniques or brain enhancement technologies, can definitely deliver intelligence-boosting effects.

Certainly, you need some natural aptitude to excel in most facets of life – be it mental, physical or artistic – but if genius was simply a matter of inheriting good genes, then many more of us would be geniuses.

Anyway, we predict, or sincerely hope, that formal education will one day be reflective of what occurs within the fictional Pedemont Orphanage of our thriller series – minus the assassination training of course!

Equally, we firmly believe some if not most of the alternative learning methods mentioned in *Genius Intelligence* will eventually become the norm for students the world over.

To return to that other awkward subject – who we are and what the hell we are doing writing about the secrets of the genius mindset. Well, that's a trickier one to satisfy readers on so early in the piece...

All we can really say is we write fiction and non-fiction books and produce movies in our dual careers as authors and filmmakers. In our earlier careers, we have between us held a variety of positions in different fields spanning the arts, media, PR and retail sectors. Those positions include journalist, bookseller, publicist and newspaper editor.

So we shall have to leave it up to you as to whether you think this book is a work of "genius" or not.

One reason we wrote this book is because, in our opinion, most other titles on the subject of increasing intelligence make for disappointing reading. In the main, they are not written for the average person. They're written *for* academics *by* people with PhD's.

The end result, more often than not, are books that resemble academic text and which rarely venture beyond scientifically proven and well-established mainstream methodologies.

Paradoxical though it may sound, we are convinced that *not* being from the world of academia, or even being particularly studious, eminently qualified us to write this book. After all, we wrote it to empower the average individual – the 'common' working class person. We can relate to such people as that's exactly our background.

One thing we can promise is that after researching far and wide in some unusual and unlikely places, the pages of this book contain the most advanced accelerated learning methods available on the planet.

Wishing you well on your path to increasing your IQ!

James Morcan & Lance Morcan

1

GENIUS TECHNIQUES OF THE ELITE

It has long been speculated that secret societies, mystery schools, intelligence agencies and other clandestine organizations have advanced learning methods superior to anything taught in even the most prestigious universities. Methods which are only ever taught to the chosen few – initiates who have all sworn an oath to keep the group's syllabus *in house* and never reveal any of the teachings to outsiders.

On the rare occasions the public get wind of these types of advanced learning techniques – usually via information leaked to the Internet, sometimes via published books – they are seldom tested or given the attention they deserve and so largely remain in obscurity. One reason for this could be the advanced techniques are often not comprehensible because whoever is behind them has withheld the overall curriculum.

There's many a tale of mysterious figures from secretive groups mastering skills, languages and even complex career paths so quickly that most would say it's impossible.

But that opinion assumes we common people know of, or have access to, all the learning methods known to man.

If we are to assume there are superior learning methods not taught in our mainstream education system then this naturally leads to other questions.

What if your child's top-notch education is actually a second-rate education?

Or, if you are a student, what if that professor you look up to is no mastermind, but just a tool of an inferior learning institution?

None of this is to disrespect formal education. It plays a vital role in society and the betterment of Mankind, and only a fool would doubt the importance of getting a good education.

Nor are we suggesting there isn't the odd learning institution that teaches at least some accelerated learning techniques, although such establishments would probably exist on the fringes of mainstream education.

The Montessori system is possibly one such example as it allows children to have greater freedom of expression and to learn in playful and organic ways.

Successful alumni of the Montessori education system include Amazon founder Jeff Bezos, Nobel Prize-winning author Gabriel García Márquez, Wikipedia founder Jimmy Wales, tennis champion Roger Federer (Figure 4) and Google co-founders Sergey Brin and Larry Page.

In general, however, accelerated learning methods are more likely to be found outside the modern education system.

Let's face it, wherever in the world you go, real prodigies are the exception not the norm in the present system. Those rare individuals whom society labels as geniuses are almost always *freaks of nature* and are *naturally gifted* rather than being diligent students who became geniuses as a result of their education.

"I'll be a genius and the world will admire me. Perhaps I'll be despised and misunderstood, but I'll be a genius, a great genius."

~ Salvador Dalí.
Written in his diary at the age of 16.

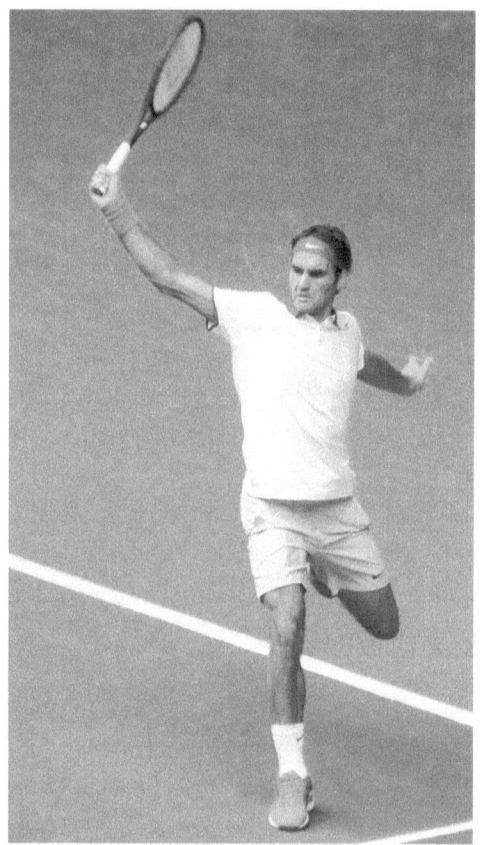

Figure 4: Roger Federer... Montessori alumni

"R Federer Australian Open 2014"
by Peter Myers from Melbourne, Australia

Federer - Oz Open 2014. Licensed under CC BY 2.0 via Wikimedia
Commons

2

POLYMATHS AND HIGH-IQ INDIVIDUALS

"The purpose of having the orphans study all these diverse fields was not for them to just become geniuses, but to become polymaths – meaning they would be geniuses in a wide variety of fields. Whether they were studying the sciences, languages, international finance, politics, the arts or martial arts, they would not stop until they'd achieved complete mastery of that subject. Kentbridge himself had encyclopedic knowledge about almost everything, and expected nothing less from his orphans."

~ The Ninth Orphan

A book critic who reviewed *The Ninth Orphan*, book one in our thriller series, criticized our protagonist Nine (the ninth-born orphan) for having an IQ, or intelligence quotient, higher than Einstein's. The strong implication in the review was that this was a ridiculous character decision we, the authors, had made.

That all sounds like a valid criticism on the surface, but had this critic gone beyond his own sphere of knowledge and done a little research he would have discovered there are many people whose IQ's have been recorded to be higher than Einstein's.

American author Marilyn Vos Savant, for example, has an IQ of 192; Russian chess grandmaster and former world champion Garry Kasparov has an IQ of 194. Incidentally, Einstein's IQ was estimated in the 1920's to between 160 and 190.

But wait, there's much more when it comes to the world of super geniuses…

Quite a few individuals have tested in excess of a 200 IQ score, including South Korean civil engineer Kim Ung-yong (210), former child prodigy and NASA employee Christopher Hirata (225) and Australian mathematician Terence Tao (225-230).

And last but not least is American child prodigy, mathematician and politician William James Sidis who had an IQ of 250-300 (Figure 5). He graduated grammar school at age six, he went to Harvard University at age 11 and graduated *cum laude* at the age of 16. Sidis, who died in 1944, could fluently speak 40 languages by the time he reached adulthood.

According to the book *IQ and the Wealth of Nations*, by Dr. Richard Lynn and Dr. Tatu Vanhanen, the top five countries in terms of average IQ's of their citizens are Hong Kong (107), South Korea (106), Japan (105), Taiwan (104) and Singapore (103). Further down the list, China, New Zealand and the UK share equal 12th position with a 100 average, while the US is in 19th position with an average citizen IQ of 98.

However, many scholars in the 21st Century now believe IQ scores aren't everything and it's likely areas of intelligence exist that cannot be measured in any test. This is possibly substantiated by the number of successful and iconic individuals who recorded very low IQ scores. These include the once highly articulate and outspoken boxer Muhammad Ali who, as a young man, scored only 78 – an IQ so low it supposedly denotes a mild mental disability!

And of course, the list of the world's so-called most intelligent *excludes* extremely bright individuals in impoverished parts of the world where IQ's are, or were, rarely tested. The Indian mathematical genius, Srinivasa Ramanujan (1887-1920), was an example of such incredible geniuses who defy all explanation.

You'll recall Dr. Takaaki Musha refers to Ramanujan in the Foreword, mentioning how he was inspired by the gentleman's advanced mathematical findings.

Born into poverty in Erode, India, Ramanujan discovered extraordinary mathematical formulas despite being self-taught with no formal training in mathematics. He changed the face of mathematics as we know it and left many highly-educated and acclaimed Western mathematicians completely gobsmacked.

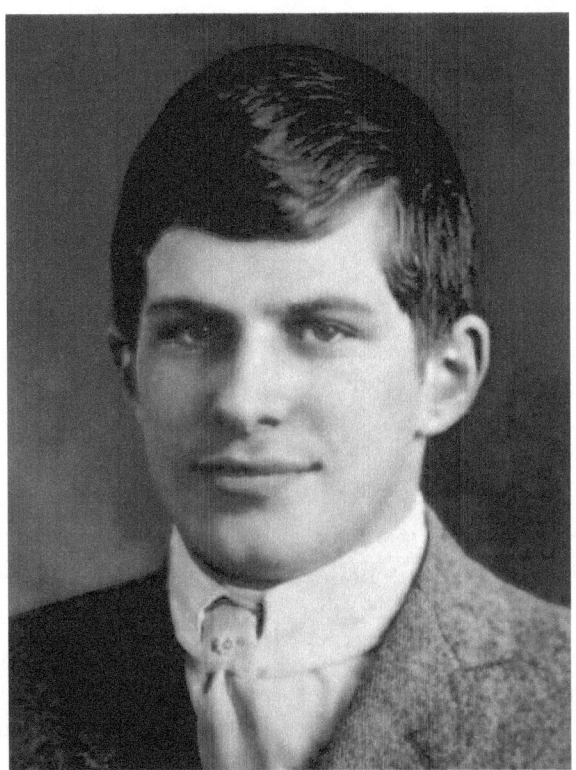

Figure 5: *Sidis... 20th Century child prodigy*

"William James Sidis 1914" by Unknown - The Sidis Archives.

Licensed under Public Domain via Wikimedia Commons

Furthermore, the other high-IQ individuals mentioned earlier are only in the top bracket of those who *agreed* to undergo IQ tests *and* allow their scores to be published.

It's quite conceivable certain elite individuals belonging to secret societies, mystery schools or intelligence agencies do not reveal their IQ scores. That secret intelligence factor was the basis for our fictional Pedemont orphans in *The Orphan Trilogy* whom we either state or imply have IQ's of around 200 or higher.

As a result of the accelerated learning techniques within the diverse curriculum that begins before they can even walk or talk, the orphans can assimilate and retain phenomenal amounts of information. By their teens, the child prodigies are more knowledgeable even than adult geniuses. They can solve complex problems, are fully knowledgeable about almost any current world subject or historical event, and are to all intents and purposes organic supercomputers and human library databases.

Our orphans are exposed to highly advanced learning methods so that they will have at their disposal all the necessary skills and information to be able to overcome life-and-death problems that may arise on future espionage assignments. They're taught there is no challenge or question that cannot be overcome, solved or answered as long as they fully utilize the power of their minds.

Each child at the Pedemont Orphanage eventually becomes a *polymath* – a person who is beyond a genius. It's a word we use throughout the trilogy as we felt it best describes the orphans' off-the-scale intellects.

A polymath is actually a *multiple-subject genius*. However, the criterion for a polymath is someone who is an expert in vastly different, almost unrelated fields. For example, an artist who works in the film, theatre and literary industries and who is a masterful actor, screenwriter, novelist, film director and film producer would *not* qualify as a polymath as those fields are all artistic mediums and closely related.

Rather, a polymath is someone who has excelled in, or completely mastered, a variety of unrelated or loosely related subjects. These could be as diverse as economics, dance, architecture, mathematics, history, forensic science, cooking and entomology.

And before you go calling yourself a polymath, don't forget you must be an *expert* in each field. Unfortunately being a jack-of-all-trades and master-of-none doesn't count.

One of the best examples of a polymath is Leonardo da Vinci (Figure 6).

Born in Italy in 1452, Leonardo was a sculptor, painter, architect, mathematician, musician, engineer, inventor, anatomist, botanist, geologist, cartographer and writer. Although he received an informal education that included geometry, Latin and mathematics, he was essentially an *autodidact*, or a self-taught individual.

The man who many have called *the* most diversely talented person who ever lived, left behind an array of masterpieces in the painting world alone, including *The Last Supper*, *Mona Lisa* and *The Vitruvian Man* *(Figure 7)*.

"The knowledge of all things is possible"

~ *Leonardo da Vinci*

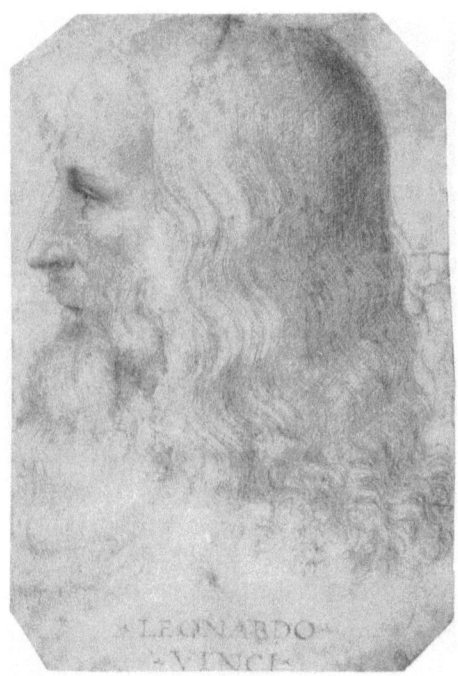

Figure 6: *Portrait of Leonardo da Vinci c. 1510*

"Francesco Melzi - Portrait of Leonardo - WGA14795" by Francesco Melzi

Web Gallery of Art. Licensed under Public Domain via Wikimedia Commons

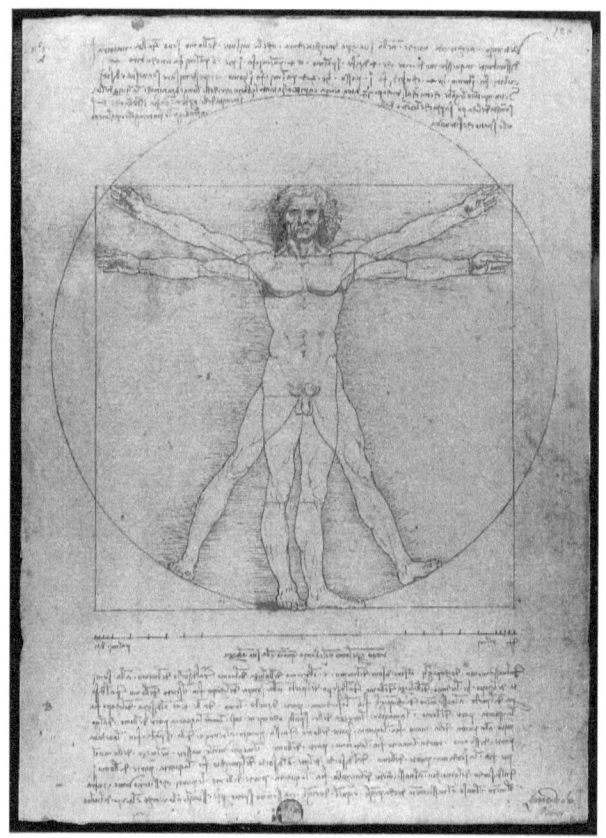

Figure 7: *Leonardo da Vinci's The Vitruvian Man*

"Da Vinci Vitruve Luc Viatour" by Leonardo da Vinci
Own work www.lucnix.be. 2007-09-08 (photograph).
Photograph: This image is the work of Luc Viatour / www.Lucnix.be

3

OUTRUNNING THE CONSCIOUS MIND

"The subconscious was always favored over the everyday conscious mind, which was considered too slow to be effective."

~ *The Orphan Factory*

Developing a genius mindset essentially comes down to two things: operating at speed and using the subconscious mind more than the conscious. This intuitive or relaxed approach to study is the polar opposite of traditional and mainstream forms of education.

Apart from some artistic subjects like music or dance, learning institutions generally require pupils to concentrate hard at all times. In other words, students have no choice but to always use their conscious minds, thereby suppressing the great reservoir of the subconscious.

When we are forced to think s-l-o-w-l-y like this our brain functions at well below optimum levels. That's why school students often feel exhausted as studying in this fashion is incredibly draining.

But how can we feel mentally drained when neuroscientists and brain researchers agree we each only use a tiny percentage of our brain?

In *The Orphan Trilogy*, our orphans often go into a daydream state whenever they need answers to life-and-death situations. This is because when you defocus you allow your intuitive self, or your subconscious mind, to *deliver* the answers you need. It just happens, without reaching for it.

We've all experienced pondering a problem all day long only to find we *receive* the solution when forgetting about the problem and thinking of something else. When we stop concentrating so hard, we allow our subconscious to flourish, and those who do this more than others are sometimes called geniuses.

As head of the Pedemont Orphanage, Tommy Kentbridge says to his students in *The Orphan Factory*, "The subconscious mind is where all higher intelligences exist. Every genius throughout history – Tesla, Einstein, Da Vinci – tapped into the infinite power of their subconscious minds."

Studies have shown the subconscious mind can process around 11 million bits of information per second. The conscious mind, however, can only process about 15 to 16 bits of information per second.

Quite a difference!

One of the best ways to bring the subconscious mind into the equation is to *outrun* the conscious mind by going so fast it literally can't keep up. So, at Chicago's Pedemont Orphanage, our orphans do everything at speed. They're also taught how to learn things indirectly instead of directly. By skirting around the edges of complex subjects, the children never get information overload or lose their way.

As we wrote in *The Ninth Orphan*, "In the tradition of Leonardo da Vinci and history's other great polymaths, the children were taught how to fully understand anything by using an advanced mental technique where they would simply *life* their minds into comprehension."

To life your mind into comprehension is once again the polar opposite of modern education systems which imply there's only one way to learn: consciously and with intense concentration.

While this indirect way of learning may sound flaky, it is actually backed up by hard science and is not remotely mystical. This approach is about brainwaves and understanding, or recognizing, the optimal state for learning.

When you hit the right groove, it's possible to learn quickly and in a satisfying, even enjoyable, fashion.

It is that singularity of mind top sportsmen and martial arts masters achieve. Psychologists sometimes refer to this ultimate mental state as *the zone*, but it's really just about having the most effective brainwaves for learning.

Any time study feels laborious the student is most likely in the beta brainwave, which occurs when the conscious mind is governing. A beta-dominant mind is the perfect recipe for mediocrity and boredom.

The subconscious mind comes into play in other less common brainwaves such as alpha, gamma, theta and delta. These brainwaves have also been shown to be activated when test subjects are laughing, daydreaming, meditating, singing, dancing or spontaneously moving about.

Now how many math or English teachers would tolerate those activities in their classrooms?

What if there really is a much quicker, less methodical way of learning that allows you to learn without learning?

Sounds paradoxical, doesn't it?

"Talent hits a target no one else can hit. Genius hits a target no one else can see."

~ Arthur Schopenhauer

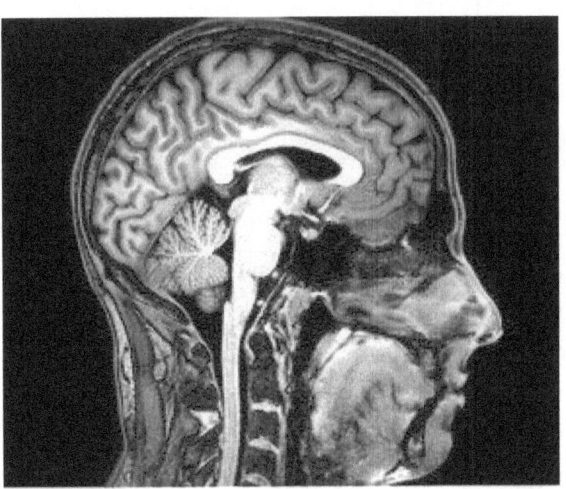

Figure 8: *A high quality T3 fMRI brain scan*

"FMRI Brain Scan" by DrOONeil - Own work.
Licensed under CC BY-SA 3.0 via Wikimedia Commons

OTHER BOOKS BY LANCE & JAMES MORCAN

published by Sterling Gate Books

Historical Fiction:

White Spirit (A novel based on a true story)
Into the Americas (A novel based on a true story)
World Odyssey (The World Duology, #1)
Fiji: A Novel (The World Duology, #2)

Conspiracy Thrillers:

The Ninth Orphan (The Orphan Trilogy, #1)
The Orphan Factory (The Orphan Trilogy, #2)
The Orphan Uprising (The Orphan Trilogy, #3)

Crime Thrillers:

Silent Fear (A novel inspired by true crimes)
The Heathrow Affair
The Me Too Girl

Action-Adventure:

The Dogon Initiative
High Country Contract

Non-Fiction:

DEBUNKING HOLOCAUST DENIAL THEORIES:
Two Non-Jews Affirm the Historicity of the Nazi Genocide

THE ORPHAN CONSPIRACIES:
29 Conspiracy Theories from The Orphan Trilogy

GENIUS INTELLIGENCE:
Secret Techniques and Technologies to Increase IQ
(The Underground Knowledge Series, #1)

ANTIGRAVITY PROPULSION:
Human or Alien Technologies?
(The Underground Knowledge Series, #2)

MEDICAL INDUSTRIAL COMPLEX:
The $ickness Industry, Big Pharma and Suppressed Cures
(The Underground Knowledge Series, #3)

THE CATCHER IN THE RYE ENIGMA:
J.D. Salinger's Mind Control Triggering Device or a Coincidental
Literary Obsession of Criminals?
(The Underground Knowledge Series, #4)

INTERNATIONAL BANKSTER$:
The Global Banking Elite Exposed and the Case for Restructuring
Capitalism
(The Underground Knowledge Series, #5)

BANKRUPTING THE THIRD WORLD:
How the Global Elite Drown Poor Nations in a Sea of Debt
(The Underground Knowledge Series, #6)

UNDERGROUND BASES:
Subterranean Military Facilities and the Cities Beneath Our Feet
(The Underground Knowledge Series, #7)

Short Stories by Lance Morcan

5 SHORT STORY GEMS:
Once Were Brothers / Mr. 100% / A Gladiator's Love / The Last
Tasmanian Tiger / Brooklyn Bankster

www.ingramcontent.com/pod-product-compliance
Lightning Source LLC
Chambersburg PA
CBHW030647220526
45463CB00005B/1666